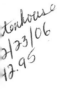

Applied Ethics
in Nursing

* * * * * * * * * * * * *

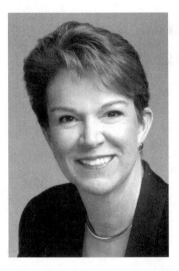

Vicki D. Lachman, PhD, MBE, APRN, is an Associate Professor in the College of Nursing at Drexel University, Philadelphia. In her role at the university and as a national consultant, she primarily teaches ethics, leadership and psychiatry. She is known for her practical, dynamic, and thought-provoking presentations. Dr. Lachman has over 30 years of experience as a psychotherapist and an organizational development consultant. Since receiving her master's degree in Bioethics from the University of Pennsylvania in 2002, she has added advising executives on organizational ethics and front-line staff on end-of-life ethical issues.

Applied Ethics
in Nursing

* * * * * * * * * * *

Vicki D. Lachman, PhD, MBE, APRN

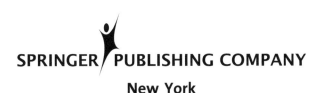

SPRINGER PUBLISHING COMPANY

New York

Springer Publishing Company, Inc.
11 West 42nd Street
New York, NY 10036-8002

Acquisitions Editor: Ruth Chasek
Production Editor: Jeanne Libby
Cover design by Joanne Honigman
Typeset by International Graphic Services, Inc., Newtown, PA

06 07 08 09 10 / 5 4 3 2 1

Library of Congress Cataloging-in-Publication Data

Applied ethics in nursing / [edited by] Vicki D. Lachman.
    p. ; cm.
Includes bibliographical references and index.
ISBN 0-8261-7984-3
1. Nursing ethics.   I. Lachman, Vicki D.
[DNLM: 1. Ethics, Nursing.   WY 85 A649 2006]
RT85.A674 2006
174.2—dc22
2005026321

Printed in the United States of America by Bang Printing.

Contents

Contributors

Deborah Antai-Otong, MS, APRN, BC, FAAN
Acting Program Coordinator
Veterans Integrated Systems
  Network (VISN) 17
Care Coordination Home
  Telehealth
Arlington, TX

Julia W. Aucoin, DNS, RN, BC
Assistant Professor
University of North Carolina at
  Greensboro
Greensboro, NC

Joyce Bedoian, MBE, MSN, RN, CRNP
Coordinator Nursing Learning
  Resource Center
Widener University School of
  Nursing
Chester, PA

Syvil S. Burke, MSN, MBA, RN
Associate Operating Officer
Duke University Hospital
Durham, NC

Caroline Camuñas, EdD, RN
Adjunct Associate Professor
Teachers College
Columbia University
New York and Veterans Affairs
  Medical Center
New York, NY

Ursula H. Capewell, MSN, RN, CT, CSA
Health Educator
Duke University Health System
Durham, NC

Doris V. Chaplin, MN, RN
Instructor
Midlands Technical College
Columbia, SC

Michael Dahnke, PhD
Independent Scholar and Adjunct
  Instructor
The College of New Jersey
Ewing, NJ
St. Joseph's University and Drexel
  University
Philadelphia, PA

Susan B. Dickey, PhD, RN
Associate Professor
Temple University
Philadelphia, PA

H. Michael Dreher, DNSc, RN
Associate Professor and Director
Doctoral Nursing Programs
Drexel University
Philadelphia, PA

Mary English Worth, CRNP, MSN
Practice consultant/private
  infertility counseling practice
West Chester, PA

Ellen Giarelli, EdD, RN, CRNP
Research Assistant Professor
University of Pennsylvania
School of Nursing
Philadelphia, PA

Dale Halsey Lea, MPH, RN, APNG, FAAN
Director, Division of Genetics
Foundation for Blood Research
Scarborough, ME

Mary Lou Helfrich Jones, PhD, RN, CNAA
Director, Subspecialty Outreach
  Programs
Clinical Contract Services,
  Business Development
International Programs
Duke University Health System
  Network Services
Durham, NC

Shirley L. Jones, PhD, RNC
Healthcare Consultant
Prospect, KY

Judith A. Lewis, PhD, RNC, FAAN
Professor, School of Nursing
Virginia Commonwealth University
Richmond, VA

Anne M. Lovell, MSN, RN, CPNP
Clinical Nurse Specialist
Division of Patient Services and
  Division of Human Genetics
Cincinnati Children's Hospital
  Medical Center
Cincinnati, OH

Margaret M. Mahon, PhD, RN, FAAN
Associate Professor
College of Nursing and Health
  Science
George Mason University
Fairfax, VA
Senior Fellow
University of Pennsylvania Center
  for Bioethics
Philadelphia, PA

Kathy Malloch, PhD, MBA, RN, FAAN
President, Kathy Malloch
  Associates
Glendale, AZ
Faculty, Arizona State University,
  College of Nursing
Tempe, AZ
Evidence Based Researcher,
  Banner Estrella Medical Center
Phoenix, AZ

Terri L. Maxwell, MSN, APRN, BC-PCM
Director of Research
excelleRx, Inc.
Philadelphia, PA

Lauren G. McAliley, MSN, MA, CNP
Assistant Director, Center for Pediatric Ethics
Rainbow Babies & Children's Hospital of University Hospitals of Cleveland
Cleveland, OH

Carolyn H. McGrory, MS, RN
Research Coordinator for the National Transplantation Pregnancy Registry
Temple University
Philadelphia, PA

Moni McIntyre, CAPT USNR, PhD
Assistant Professor
Graduate Center for Social and Public Policy
Duquesne University
Pittsburgh, PA

Eileen Mieras Kohlenberg, PhD, RN, CNAA, BC
Associate Dean and Director of Graduate Study
University of North Carolina at Greensboro
Greensboro, NC

Rose H. Mueller, BSN, RN, OCN
Director, Oncology Services
Chestnut Hill Health System
Philadelphia, PA

Sally J. Nunn, RN
Director, Clinical Outreach & Faculty Associate
Center for Bioethics
University of Pennsylvania
Philadelphia, PA

Barbara B. Ott, PhD, RN
Associate Professor
College of Nursing
Villanova University
Villanova, PA

Diane E. Radvansky, MSN, CRNP
Nurse Practitioner, Immunodeficiency Department
Albert Einstein Medical Center
Philadelphia, PA

JoAnne Reifsnyder, PhD, APRN, BC-PCM
Co-Founder, Ethos Consulting
Mt. Laurel, NJ
Assistant Professor
University of Pennsylvania
School of Nursing
Philadelphia, PA

Cindy Stern, RN, MSN, CCRP
Cancer Network Administrator
Cancer Network of the Abramson Cancer Center
University of Pennsylvania Health System
Philadelphia, PA

Diane Stillman, MSN, RN
Consultant
University of Pennsylvania
School of Nursing
Philadelphia, PA

Catherine S. Taylor, MSN, RN, BC
Coordinator
Patient/Family and Community
  Education
Duke University Health System
Durham, NC

Martha Turner, Col USAF NC, PhD, RN, BC, CNAA
Program Director, International
  Health
Uniformed Services University
Bethesda, MD

Linda Wright, MHSc, MSW, RSW
Bioethicist
University Health Network & Joint
  Centre for Bioethics
University of Toronto
Toronto, Ontario, Canada

Preface

Applied Ethics in Nursing is designed to give practicing and student nurses an easily understandable guide to the kind of everyday ethical dilemmas they may face. The book uses a question and answer format along with numerous case studies to present best practices and strategies for approaching the difficult problems commonly found in clinical practice. It also addresses organizational and institutional issues that can confound or promote ethically sound decision making. The question-and-answer and case study format is used so that ethics is discussed in the context of "real-life" situations. Each chapter ends with a resource list of websites and recommendations for further reading. The American Nurses' Association *Code of Ethics for Nurses* is used as a guide throughout, along with standards and guidelines from other major health care and governmental organizations.

Chapter authors were selected for their expertise in their respective specialties and a knowledge of typical ethical problems found in these areas. They derived the questions and cases for their chapters from three methods. In some cases, they conducted focus groups with clinical nurses to develop situations commonly encountered. Authors also searched the literature to determine the most often discussed issues. Finally, authors worked with other experts in their field to determine the key information needed by practicing nurses in that specialty. Most chapters were developed with a combination of these three methods.

The book is divided into six parts. After establishing basic principles of ethics in Part I, a developmental perspective is used for Parts II through IV, in which ethics is presented in terms of specific life stages, from pre-conception and the beginning of life to end-of-life issues. Vulnerable populations with special ethical considerations, such as individuals with HIV/AIDS or mental illness, are included in Part III. Part V discusses developing an organizational culture that supports ethical behavior. Part VI examines specific responses of patients from different cultures and religions.

Some of the ethical issues and practical strategies for action in this book include:

- What exactly are "patient's rights" and how do you advocate for your patient?

- What is "informed consent"? What can I do if the patient lacks the capacity to make decisions?

- What is the rationale for giving a patient medication (chemical restraints) against his or her will?

- Do healthcare workers have the autonomy to refuse to care for HIV-positive patients if they believe their safety is at risk?

- How should staff handle refusal of treatment, whether it is refusal of medications or even refusal of personal care?

- Is there an internationally accepted definition of death?

- Is it ethical to ask a family to donate a loved one's organs when they have just been traumatized by the potential donor's death?

- What should a nurse do when physicians avoid approaching a family with a patient who has a poor prognosis?

- How should I respond to a patient who requests my help in dying?

- How should a professional nurse manage a situation when a colleague/peer delivers substandard care?

- What is the role of the ethics committee?

I hope you find *Applied Ethics in Nursing* an enjoyable book to read and a reference book you will turn to repeatedly. This down-to-earth, practical approach should help you manage ethical issues in an array of clinical settings, as well as provide you with strategies to manage organizational and cultural problems. I believe this book provides you with the needed guidance you desire.

Vicki D. Lachman, PhD, MBE, APRN

Part 1

The Essence of Ethics and Advocacy in Nursing

Part 1 begins with an overview of moral reasoning and the application of ethical theories to nursing practice. Understanding advocacy responsibilities and needed skills is followed by a focus on the importance of the nurses' support in the informed consent process. The chapter on Patients' Rights examines the multiple documents on this subject, as well as typical rights issues nurses confront. Finally, Part 2 ends with the application of these skills in the arena of research on human subjects.

Chapter 1

Defining Ethics and Applying the Theories

Michael Dahnke and H. Michael Dreher

1. What is ethics, and why do nurses need to understand it?

"Ethics" is commonly defined as the philosophical study of right action and wrong action, also known as "morality." Being "philosophical" does not mean that ethics is a study of or concern only to philosophers. Any human being at one point in his/her life has pondered questions of right and wrong.

It would be helpful for a nurse to understand ethics because nurses encounter many of the same ethical problems and questions as any human being. However, beyond that, because of the nature of their work, there are specific moral questions and problems that arise: questions of confidentiality, patient rights, questions of life and death. An understanding of ethics can help a nurse get a clearer view in these difficult cases of the issue at hand, the possible courses of action, and the principles underlying right action.

2. When ethics and the law appear to be in conflict, which is more important for the nurse to follow?

This is a very complicated question with no single answer. The law and ethics are not the same but often overlap and both should be taken into account in making difficult decisions. Law describes the minimum standards of acceptable behavior. Ethics delineates the highest moral standards of behavior. One might say, however, that morality is broader and hence more primary. The law does not specifically encourage us to act morally. However, many philosophers believe there is, or should be, a moral basis to the law and that we have a *prima facie* moral obligation to follow the law.

3. What does it mean to have a *prima facie* moral obligation to follow the law?

Prima facie is Latin for "at first sight," meaning in this context, "evident or true absent any further considerations." That is, some moral or legal obligations may be overridden by more pressing or important (overriding) obligations. For example, a *prima facie* moral obligation to follow the law means that in a presumptively just society laws are presumed right, proper, and good for the society. However, they are not absolute and, under the right conditions, can be overridden by concerns that are more important. Such a conflict, then, may present us with a kind of ethical dilemma.

For example, this Registered Nurse author faced such an ethical dilemma when caring for a critically ill elderly patient in the CCU years ago. When this patient suddenly arrested, the code response team had a *prima facie* legal obligation to resuscitate him, as he had "full code" status. However, the wife was in the room at the time of the cardiac arrest and she threw herself on top of her husband as the code team entered the room, begging them to "let her husband go in peace."

4. What does the term "ethical dilemma" mean?

A dilemma is defined as a problem that confronts one with a choice between options that seem or are equally unfavorable. For example, in the case of a patient in a persistent vegetative state one might face the decision between prolonging what appears to be a life with no "quality" and little or no reasonable hope of recovery, and allowing the patient to die on his/her own. This dilemma would obviously confront the physicians, the parents, and other loved ones of such a patient. However, this would be of concern for nurses also (or especially), as families often turn to nurses first for help and comfort in such situations.

5. What is the difference between a moral dilemma and an ethical dilemma?

The terms ethics and morality, as most people and some philosophers use them, are generally synonymous. However, there are philosophers who distinguish between ethics and morality, using "morality" to designate the conventional beliefs that a particular society holds and "ethics" to refer to the rational study of beliefs in general. This distinction allows us to refer to a problem as a moral dilemma but recognize a possible, reflective ethical resolution to it. An "ethical dilemma" then might be considered a higher order problem on a more theoretical, less practical, level.

6. What is the process a nurse should use to resolve a moral dilemma?

It is possible many moral dilemmas will never be fully resolved, but there are methods for coming to a clearer and deeper understanding of the issues at hand. Once this depth and clarity is achieved, an answer may present itself that is not perfect or ideal, but more considered and possibly less undesirable. Let us examine the ethical dilemma surrounding the wife and her husband's code status.

In this case, with the patient in obvious cardiac arrest, there was no time to convene a full ethics board review. The primary care RN did inform the responding MD that the patient was critically ill, had a "full code" status, and the wife was the sole legal representative. The team was obviously in a quandary about whether to literally peel the wife off her husband's body and resuscitate him or to adhere to her wishes. In this case, the primary care RN quickly contemplated the many possible outcomes. What if the patient died and the wife recanted her story? What if her attorney said she was under duress, not using sound judgment, and we had a *prima facie* legal obligation to resuscitate him? What if the wife reported the primary care RN to the State Board of Nursing?

On the other hand, what if suddenly adhering to her request was indeed the most moral action to take and the most humane? With little time to spare, the entire code team looked to the primary care RN for guidance, as this RN and the responding MD had the most to risk in this situation. Still weighing the pros and cons and the risks and benefits (albeit quickly), the primary care RN decided to follow the wife's sudden request. He suggested the responding MD quickly write a "no code" on the patient's chart, and then come back and pronounce the man. The entire code team looked at each other, not knowing really what to do next, and then the nursing supervisor and responding MD concurred. As Pastoral Care arrived, the patient died in peace, was pronounced, and no party took further action. The dilemma was resolved.

7. How does the nurse know if he/she is using good moral reasoning?

As you practice moral reasoning, you will see for yourself issues becoming clearer and the distinction between clear and fuzzy reasoning becoming more evident. This is not very different from the phenomenon in which the study of basic arithmetic aids one in eventually understanding higher mathematics. However, moral reasoning rarely if ever provides as clear and unequivocal an answer as mathematics usually does.

In the above case, the primary care RN did know that while adhering to the wife's request had real risks, it was the right thing to do. The primary care RN also had support, as the entire code team also agreed to not resuscitate the patient and let him die peacefully. In this case, the entire team probably thought they had used "good moral reasoning."

8. What is the purpose of a professional moral code like the American Nurses Association (ANA) (2001) *Code of Ethics for Nurses?*

Considering the great deal of time and thought that members of the profession invested in the development of this code, a nurse should approach it with a presumption of moral correctness. That is, presume that there is guidance and wisdom to be found within. But remember, these codes are not to be blindly followed but are meant to assist in making decisions, not as a manual to be consulted for easy answers. Countless atrocities have occurred throughout history because individuals blindly followed rules and then used those rules in order to deflect moral responsibility later.

The *Code* is an ethical standard and delineates the ethical obligations of all nurses. It provides a framework for ethical analysis and decision. If the nurse cannot in good conscience abide by the provisions of the *Code*, he/she needs to seek guidance. It is a dynamic document, so as changes occur in the social context, so may the *Code* change. It is a document that demands of the professional nurse to think critically and to honor autonomy of self and of patients. The principle of autonomy implies at least two distinct claims:

1. The autonomous individual deserves respect as a rational person capable of making his/her own decisions, and, thus, should be allowed to do so.

2. Since the autonomous individual can make her/his own decisions, he/she is responsible for those decisions. By practicing good moral reasoning, you are cultivating autonomy.

9. Is it possible to have right and wrong answers using moral reasoning?

It is true that there is a significant subjective element to morality, but one can also use objective elements when rationally attempting to solve a moral or ethical dilemma. Moral philosophers distinguish between descriptive statements that establish the facts of a case and normative statements that determine values. Obviously, descriptive statements have a primarily objective nature and, thus, are subject to rational determination. But even values, which are much more subjective than facts, can be subject to some degree of rational consideration if we determine what results might flow from those values.

One example of this is an individual nurse's belief about assisted suicide. One nurse might have a religious belief that this act is always wrong. A non-religious nurse might believe the act may have real merit in special cases. Nevertheless, this act is illegal in 49 of 50 states in the US and even the Oregon law does not allow any nursing participation in this procedure. Therefore, it may be perfectly fine for a nurse to be sympathetic to a patient's request, but the act would have serious legal consequences in all 50 states. In this case the question remains whether complicity here is morally wrong, regardless of the legal implications.

10. What is the role of religion in answering moral questions?

Religion is a guide for morality for many people. There is nothing inherently wrong in this approach to morality, but it does have its limitations. First, in a multicultural society it would be unreasonable to expect everyone to share your religious and, hence, moral convictions. Applying such a morality in a public setting can lead to a form of imposing one's beliefs (religious/moral) upon others who may have equally as strongly held religious/moral beliefs and are under no obligation to accept yours, which may clearly lead to ethical dilemmas. More importantly, since most religions establish moral principles in a dogmatic, commandment-like form, there usually is no room left for rational consideration. Thus, when facing a dilemma most religious morality may be found lacking the proper intellectual tools for handling these "hard cases."

11. What is "ethics of care"?

Ethics of care is a recently developed moral theory originally based on the insights of moral psychologist Carol Gilligan who claimed that women understand ethics differently from men. The philosophers who developed the theory rejected the traditional male-centered ethics that focused on rationality, individuality, and abstract principles in favor of emotion, caring relationships, and concrete situations. Philosopher Nel Noddings sees caring ethics as reflecting an image of human connectedness. She described personal relations as "ontologically basic and the caring relation as ethically basic" (Noddings, 1984, p. 3). In caring for others, we aspire to be our highest self.

Some in the field of nursing ethics have suggested this theory as particularly suited for nursing, but others find this theory problematic. Kuhse and Singer (2001), for example, in criticism of the theory warned that an ethics focusing entirely on the nurse/patient caring relationship risks the perpetuation of stereotypes, unequal gender roles, and oppressive, even abusive, "caring" relationships. These authors also claimed that the theory risks the loss of the nurse's moral voice (on the behalf of the nurses themselves as well as the patients), that the subjective nature of the theory does not allow for universally accessible moral principles, and that it neglects potentially important moral principles like justice.

Gilligan's "ethics of care" also raises questions about the ability of male nurses to care. Do male nurses care "more" than men do in general, or do they care differently than most men because they have been socialized to "nurse"? Alternatively, do male nurses "not care" differently from men in general?

12. What is utilitarianism and how would I use this theory in practice?

The guiding principle of utilitarianism is what is called the "principle of utility" or the "greatest happiness principle": those actions are to be chosen which will produce the greatest amount of happiness for the greatest number of people. The concept of triage is based upon this form of thinking: doling out limited resources (e.g., time, medication) based on greatest need and a capacity to benefit from the resources. When faced with a decision which will result in pain and/or pleasure (those are the elements that comprise the utilitarian understanding of happiness), a nurse could be justified in choosing the alternative that results in the greatest amount of pleasure or least amount of pain. A utilitarian approach can also be seen in the ANA (2001) *Code*'s stated purpose as "an expression of nursing's own understanding of its commitment to society" (p. 5).

13. What is pragmatism and how does it differ from utilitarianism?

Pragmatism is an American school of philosophy that rejects the esoteric metaphysics of traditional European academic philosophy in favor of more down-to-earth, concrete questions and answers. Pragmatist philosopher John Dewey developed a method of moral problem solving based on the scientific method, which very closely resembles the nursing process. Pragmatists contend the only reason people have for calling one view true and the other false is that one works in the human experience and the other does not. Miller and colleagues (1997) have adapted this method for clinical ethics into a four-step process:

1. Assessment

2. Moral diagnosis

3. Goal setting, decision making, and implementation

4. Evaluation

First, assess the facts of the situation; second, diagnose the moral problem; third, set goals and decide on a plan of action, which is then implemented; fourth, evaluate the results. Rather than allowing oneself to get caught up in esoteric quandaries of moral theory, this method provides a clear, straightforward, even democratic, approach to moral problem solving that may not always result in clear, unequivocal answers but increases the likelihood of clarifying the situation and achieving a resolution. Pragmatists believe we are in a continuous quest for workable solutions to difficulties.

14. What is deontology and what does it have to do with ethics and nursing?

Deontology is an approach to ethics that focuses on "duty," which, in fact, is what the Greek word "deon" means. Deontology is often contrasted with consequentialism, which judges actions from their consequences, not from the intent of the action. Immanuel Kant was the major proponent of deontology. In differentiating a moral action from an immoral one, a good person acts from a sense of duty, not from inclinations and feelings. An individual would repay debts not to avoid punishment but because it is the right thing to do.

For example, a nurse might attempt to justify informing the spouse of a patient with a communicable disease against the patient's wishes in order to prevent cross-infection of the spouse. The nurse has a duty to protect the patient's confidentiality and also a duty to protect the public. She would need to inform the patient of her duty to report (mandated by state). She should also encourage the patient to discuss it with his/her spouse.

Provision 2 of the ANA (2001) *Code* defines the nurse's paramount duty as commitment to the patient. Section 2.2 states, "Nurses . . . must seek to ensure that employment arrangements are just and fair and do not create unreasonable conflict between patient care and direct personal gain" (p. 10), which outlines a sense of duty that places the patient first, ahead of a nurse's personal gain.

15. What is virtue theory?

Virtue theory is the ethical theory probably least used in the consideration of professional or applied ethics, which is unfortunate. The reason for applied ethics' general neglect of it is probably that unlike deontological theories or consequentialist theories, virtue theory is not geared toward answering specific questions, or making specific ethical decisions. Rather, virtue theory, as originally developed by the philosopher Aristotle, aims toward the cultivation of good character. If one learns and practices virtues (e.g., honesty, courage), one will develop good character from which will flow good actions and good decisions. The cultivation of good character would be valuable to nurses as they grow themselves within their profession. If they work to instill virtues within themselves, good actions and decisions are more likely to follow. If they fail to do this, sloppy thinking and ill-considered decisions are likely to follow. Aristotle based his choice of proper virtues on those that tend toward the proper good of "man." We can appropriate this way of thinking and determine that the proper virtues of nurses are those that will tend to create the best nurses.

16. What does the term bioethics actually mean?

Bioethics is the subdiscipline of applied ethics that studies the moral questions surrounding biology, medicine, and the health professions in general. It is a term sometimes used interchangeably with "medical ethics," but more appropriately, bioethics is a broader category that would include medical ethics. The issues explored by bioethicists include questions of research ethics: the use of patients in clinical drug trials, stem cell research, human cloning; questions of medical ethics: patient autonomy, euthanasia, abortion, gene therapy, and broader social questions: genetic testing, the role of physicians in society, the commercialization of health care. This, of course, is not a complete list, but merely a sampling of the many issues and questions addressed in the study of bioethics.

17. What does the term justice mean?

Harvard philosopher John Rawls (2001) provided a brief definition of justice in one of his works: "the elimination of arbitrary distinctions and the establishment within the structure of a practice of a proper share, balance, or equilibrium between competing claims" (p. 191). According to the concept of justice, then, there is a certain inherent rightness or wrongness in actions based on fairness in distribution. That is, someone receiving a punishment equal to the crime he/she committed is receiving a just punishment. Someone receiving back money lent out is being treated justly. Someone keeping money spewed out by a malfunctioning ATM machine, however, is being unjustly rewarded. Nurses may find themselves facing questions of the just distribution of health care, especially regarding the question of income level as an arbitrary distinction in relation to healthcare distribution.

18. What is a "right" in ethics?

A "right" is a claim someone holds, which imposes a duty upon others. For example, in the practice of nursing, most patients would probably say they have a right to unconditional care from a professional nurse. A nurse might likewise believe he/she has a right to advocate on the patient's behalf.

Rights are often described as positive or negative. "Negative" rights are rights of noninterference, meaning that all that is necessary for you to enjoy your right is for others to leave you be. "Positive" rights are rights that impose affirmative or active duties upon others. For example, if health care were seen as a positive right, then a form of universal health coverage would seem to be obligatory. If health care were seen as a negative right, one could seek out health care freely and without his/her rights violated as long as no one inhibits or prohibits him/her from doing so. Section 3 of the ANA (2001) *Code* imposes a duty upon nurses to safeguard several rights of patients: privacy, confidentiality, and self-determination.

19. How can I use ethical reasoning in my practice as a nurse?

Although the various theories may seem to conflict and even contradict, some philosophers suggest seeing them as wells we can draw from depending on the needs of the situation we find ourselves in. Utilitarianism can keep us mindful of the importance of the consequences of our actions, the effect these actions have on others, and the duty to minimize suffering. Kantian ethics can keep in front of our eyes the importance of dignity, autonomy, and responsibility. By developing the virtue of courage, we can better advocate for patients. In addition, perhaps, most directly regarding the specifics of this question, Dewey's pragmatist ethics can remind us of the constantly changing nature of the human experience, which brings with it the need for a flexible and evolving approach to ethics.

RESOURCES

American Nurses Association. (2001). *Code of ethics for nurses with interpretive statements*. Washington, DC: American Nurses Publishing.

Kuhse, H. (1997). *Caring: Nurses, women and ethics*. Malden, MA: Blackwell Publishers.

Kuhse, H., & Singer, P. (2001). *A companion to bioethics*. Malden, MA: Blackwell Publishers.

Miller, F. G., Fletcher, J. C., & Fins, J. J. (1997). Clinical pragmatism: A case method of moral problem solving. In J. C. Fletcher, P. A. Lombardo, M. F. Marshall, & F. G. Miller (Eds.), *Introduction to clinical ethics* (2nd ed., pp. 21–38). Frederick, MD: University Publishing Group.

Noddings, N. (1984). *Caring: A feminine approach to ethics and moral education*. Berkeley, CA: University of California Press.

Rawls, J. (2001). Justice as reciprocity. In S. Freeman (Ed.), *Collected papers* (pp. 190–224). Cambridge, MA: Harvard University Press.

GLOSSARY OF ETHICAL TERMS

1. AUTONOMY—right to self-determination; being one's own person without constraints by another's actions or psychological and physical limitations.

2. BENEFICENCE—duty to do good.

3. CONFIDENTIALITY—holding information entrusted in the context of special relationships as private.

4. FIDELITY—duty to keep one's promise or word.

5. GRATITUDE—duty to make up for a good; what do I owe?

6. JUSTICE—treating people fairly; equitable distribution of risks and benefits.

7. NONMALEFICENCE—duty to do no harm.

8. REPARATION—duty to make up for a wrong.

9. SANCTITY OF LIFE—the standard that life is precious. This standard is used for appraising other ethical principles. No human rights and no valuation of human life can be established without presupposing this principle.

10. UTILITY—doing the greatest good or the least harm for the greatest number of people.

11. VERACITY—truth telling or the duty to tell the truth.

Chapter 2

Knowing When and How to Advocate

Martha Turner and Moni McIntyre

1. What does having an ethical responsibility to advocate for my patients mean?

To have an ethical responsibility means to have an obligation to act as an advocate. It is not optional. The ANA (2001) *Code of Ethics* describes ethical responsibilities that arise from nursing's own understanding of its commitment to society. The origin of advocacy is the Latin word *advocatus*, which means one who is called to support another. "Advocate" is both a noun and a verb. An advocate is a person who speaks in support of another or an intercessor; to advocate is to speak or write for another or for a cause. "Advocacy" is a noun and is used in current literature to describe the process of advocating. Mallik (1997) has analyzed the nursing literature on advocacy and identified these themes: Advocacy is a traditional role for nurses; nurses are in the best position on the healthcare team to advocate; nurses know how to advocate; and nurses and patients can be partners in advocacy. Remember that others on the healthcare team are also advocates for the patient; therefore, a collaborative approach will often lighten the load.

2. Does the ANA *Code of Ethics for Nurses* tell nurses to advocate for their patients?

The *Code of Ethics for Nurses* is "a succinct statement of the ethical obligations and duties of every individual who enters the nursing profession"

(p. 5). There are nine provisions in the code, and the third one addresses advocacy. It states, "The nurse promotes, advocates for and strives to protect the health, safety and rights of the patient" (p. 12). In the interpretive statements for this third provision, nurses are asked to advocate for an environment that provides for physical privacy and auditory privacy when discussing issues of a personal nature. Other issues listed in the provision include protecting the confidentiality of the patients and protecting participants in research studies. This provision also describes the nurse's responsibility to implement and maintain standards of professional nursing practice. In the other eight provisions, advocacy is implied in many of the interpretive statements.

3. What skills do I need to be a good advocate?

The skills needed for advocacy are many of the same skills required for best nursing practice. They include attentive listening, problem solving, decision making, bargaining, negotiating, conflict resolution, perseverance, and the highly developed skills of verbal and nonverbal communication. Further understanding of the ability to be a good advocate can be gained by considering the traits described by other authors. The traits identified in the research by Chafey and colleagues (1998) are being empathetic, nurturing, ethical, objective, and assertive. Luther (2000) would add the attributes of self-awareness, open-mindedness, a broad knowledge base, self-confidence, and cultural competence. Greggs-McQuilkin (2002) stated that, in addition to being an advocate for patients, nurses are called to advocate for quality in healthcare delivery systems and for the profession itself.

4. What problems can I anticipate when I advocate for patients?

There are many barriers present in the healthcare environment that make advocating difficult. Short staffing, knowledge deficits, power differentials, fatigue, fear, and lack of support are a few of them. When you advocate for patients, sometimes you will be misunderstood, and you may be perceived as not being loyal to the institution. Some may view you as a troublemaker, and you may be reprimanded. To minimize these outcomes, you should become familiar with the organizational structure, lines of authority, job descriptions, ethics committee, grievance procedures, and disciplinary processes where you work. Use this information with your best communication skills to address problems you encounter when advocating for patients.

5. *Case:* I had a physician tell me today to "mind my own business." It was her patient and she would decide what level of pain was tolerable. What is my responsibility?

    Your responsibility is to advocate for the patient to achieve a pain level satisfactory to the patient. In this situation, advocating for the patient is also advocating for the institution since failure to treat pain is a liability issue for members of the healthcare team and for the facility. The Agency for Healthcare Research and Quality (formerly the Agency for Health Care Policy and Research) explained that the patient's self-report is the single most reliable indicator of the existence and intensity of pain. McCaffery and Pasero (1999) have explained that "pain is whatever the experiencing person says it is, existing whenever he says it does" (p. 5). It is important for you to become familiar with the policies on pain management in the institution, particularly as they relate to lines of authority and accountability for pain management. You can then refer to the assessment process to be used and the time frame for appropriate response by members of the healthcare team.

    Patients and their families should be educated on the appropriate actions to take if pain is not adequately relieved. According to the American Pain Society (1999), "The clinician must accept the patient's report of pain" (p. 3). The Joint Commission on Accreditation of Healthcare Organizations offers support by stating that patients have the right to appropriate assessment and management of pain. Reporting pain, describing the effects of pain medication, and developing a pain management plan with the provider are all actions patients and their families can take if pain is unrelieved.

    There are several strategies for discussing this with the provider. Use quotes from the patient to describe the experience from the patient's perspective. Suggest that the pain level has changed in the time that has elapsed since the provider made rounds. Explain the patient's activities and the associated pain anticipated with the additional movement.

6. **What are examples of some typical situations where I would need to advocate?**

Some of the most common situations occur when there are competing loyalties to the patient and the facility or in nurse-to-nurse conflicts or nurse-to-physician conflicts. Another common conflict is when the patient's need or desire is different from the family's. For example, your assessment should always include the reflection, "in what ways should I advocate for this patient?" Questions to help guide this reflection might include: What are the cultural considerations, if any; are there any problems with communication; any sensory deficits; or is the patient just too tired to speak up?

7.　How can I teach others to advocate?

First of all, be assured that advocacy can be learned and, like mastering any skill, it takes practice to become an expert advocate. There are at least three approaches to help your peers become better advocates. The first is to be a role model for them. Take every opportunity to recount situations where you acted as an advocate whether you were successful or not. They may have suggestions that you can use too. The next approach is staff education. Plan inservice classes on advocacy; use experts from within your facility or guest speakers from the community. You can also request that the education department present a continuing education program on advocacy skills and processes. The third approach is to observe those who work with you who are good advocates. Watch what they do and how they do it and then discuss it with your peers. That way everyone learns.

8.　How can I support/reinforce the medical treatment plan in a timely fashion when there is a lack of communication with the physician?

There are two important parts to this question. The first is supporting or reinforcing the treatment plan and the second is communicating with the physician. In order to give your support to the treatment plan, you must make sure you fully understand it and agree with it. For complete understanding, make sure you know why the treatment has been prescribed, what the expected outcomes are, and what the consequences of not participating in the treatment plan might be. If you have any questions or are uncertain about the plan being right for the patient or the patient's ability to participate in the plan, you must resolve your concerns with the physician.

When it is difficult to communicate with the physician you must determine the nature of the difficulty. Once the nature of the difficulty has been determined, adapt the interpersonal skills you already use. A useful question is, "What are the goals of care for this patient?" Some common sources of communication problems are speaking English as a second language, difficult personalities, and lack of trust, not enough time, or unclear lines of authority.

9. *Case:* **One of the pediatric patients wants her parents to visit less often so she could rest, but doesn't want to offend them by telling them to go home. What should I do/say?**

   In this situation, you can advocate for the patient by suggesting to the parents that they plan their visits around the patient's treatment and rest schedule and that they need to care for themselves by getting enough rest. You may also encourage the patient to reassure her parents that she is all right when they are not visiting.

10. **What can I do when the patient doesn't like the food that is served in the hospital?**

Supporting a patient's dietary preferences can make a big difference in the patient's comfort. Contact food services to request the help of a dietician to see if any of the preferences can be met in the facility. You could also contact the family and invite them to bring in foods that the patient might like. This is especially important if there are particular ethnic foods that are not widely/easily available.

11. **How should I approach the patient's request for extended visiting hours?**

There are several things to consider when a patient requests an extension of visiting hours. First, consider the patient's need for rest. A rest period before visitors arrive may need to be built into the schedule. Reminding the patient that rest is important may be necessary.

   Second, companionship that visitors provide can promote healing. Some cultures engage in various healing rituals at the bedside. Try to accommodate them while maintaining a healing environment for the rest of the patients. If extended visiting is possible in the facility, then find out what the "after hours" security plan is so you can inform the visitors. If policy requires permission from a supervisor to extend visiting hours, then find out who it is and how to get clearance for the visitors.

12. *Case:* **The physician said to discharge the patient to her home. She was about to be discharged when her**

husband said he couldn't care for her at home. What should I do now?

As hard as you try to make realistic discharge plans, sometimes there are last minute changes to the plan. If you have a discharge planning service, then you should contact it with the new information about the husband's abilities to care for his wife. Social workers are also good resources for this kind of problem. Another approach might be to talk to the husband about his concerns and then make referrals for those aspects of the care that will be difficult. Possible sources of help are neighbors, family members, or church communities.

13. *Case:* **After treatments in the physical therapy department many patients complain of being left alone to use the equipment. Often they don't do the exercises because they are unsure of the directions given by the therapist. Should I approach the physical therapist?**

As the patient's advocate you must approach the Physical Therapy Department to resolve this concern. Explain to the therapists that patients have questions about their therapy and you would like to understand the exercises so you can support the patients when they are back on the unit.

14. *Case:* **There is a patient on our unit who drives everybody crazy with her negative comments and criticism of the staff. What can I do to help us not develop negative behavior when caring for her?**

Being an advocate for difficult patients is a real challenge. This is one of those risky situations where you may have to confront your peers. Begin by arranging for a patient-centered conference or take time at shift report to determine a consistent plan of action. Also, decide as a group how to support each other. Taking turns in caring for the patient will prevent any one staff member from becoming worn down from the negativity.

15. How can I help patients to use Internet medical resources while ensuring credibility of source?

You can advocate for patients in their efforts to become better informed with online information by recommending reliable sites and giving them guidelines for determining the quality of the information they find. Studzinsky (2002) listed the criteria developed in 1998 by the Health Summit Working Group and the National Agency for Health Care Policy and Research for assessing quality of healthcare information. These criteria are credibility, content, disclosure, links, design, interactivity, and caveats. Using these criteria, the Health on the Net Foundation reviews health sites for compliance with basic standards. Have patients look for the Foundation Seal containing the words HON@CODE on any healthcare site.

If they appear, then it helps the patient to know the source and purpose of the data he/she is reading. Suggest that the patient print the information to facilitate discussion with the healthcare provider.

16. *Case:* **A patient does not speak up for himself when the physician changes the subject about his prognosis. What are some simple things I can teach him to be better at self-advocacy for?**

    First, it is important to establish the fact that the patient wants to know. After that, determine if the physician has more information than is being shared. If the patient desires, then help him gain access to his chart. If the patient wants more information, then consider the following steps:

    1. Have the patient make a list of questions to ask.
    2. Set up an appointment with the patient, physician, and anyone else the patient would like to attend.
    3. Encourage him to ask for clarification of any points that are unclear.
    4. Practice with him, if he would like.

17. *Case:* **I have a patient whose family wants to ask her physician for a referral to a regional hospital. The patient agrees with the suggestion. Her family will provide transportation for the appointment and any associated tests and procedures. The patient and the family members are afraid it will offend the physician if they ask for the referral. Several family members have said, "Maybe we shouldn't get involved." How can I help them?**

    Advocacy for patients and their families is well supported by several ethical principles. The principle of autonomy supports having patients make decisions about their own care. In this case, it is the decision to seek care at another facility. You can reassure the patient and her family that asking for a referral is an appropriate request. Help them make an appointment with the physician so they can sit down and discuss it rather than try for a quick hallway conversation. Another principle that supports your advocating for the patient's family is beneficence. This principle supports your engaging with the family in their effort. Help them prepare for the conversation with the physician by organizing the points they want to make and clearly articulating the plan for seeking care at the other facility. It is important that everyone involved in the patient's care is comfortable with the treatment plan and has confidence that there will be continuity if the referral is made.

18. *Case:* **In the same day surgery unit there was a delay in discharging an elderly patient following a surgical procedure. His expected discharge at 4 p.m. was postponed until 9 p.m. By then it was nightfall and his wife could not drive in the dark. The hospital policy made no provisions for overnight stays. Eventually, we got approval for the overnight stay but the policy should be changed to provide for this and other contingencies. How can I help get the policy changed?**

Advocacy for change in organizational policy is one of the greatest challenges in professional practice. The first thing to do is to identify and understand the processes for change in the organization. After talking to the nurse manager, offer to prepare a written proposal for a change in the policy. Talk to other members on the unit to see if they have had similar experiences with unexpected delays in discharging patients. Ask if there are other units in the facility where a change in policy might be useful. Identify barriers to changing the policy and address them individually in your proposal. If the problem has been identified by others and they are already working on a proposal, then join their effort. If not, start alone and recruit coworkers to help you. If you are the first, then a precedent will be set. This will make it easier for others to get policies changed. You can expect to have disagreement while developing your proposal. Take the time to resolve the conflicts because they will not go away. This is especially important for the implementation of the policy. When you make mistakes, learn from them. Before long there will be another policy you will want to change.

19. *Case:* **I'm worried that a proposed new national policy will affect patients' ability to get their prescription medications. I want to help get it defeated. Where do I start?**

This is a great example of grassroots advocacy. You will be more effective if you can partner with others who share your goals. Perhaps the state nurses' association, a specialty organization, or the ANA is already involved in attempts to defeat the policy. To find out who else is concerned with the proposed legislation ask questions, spread the word, and raise awareness about the probable consequences for patients. Carefully examine the health and social justice issues for points to support your arguments. Organize your efforts, support each other, and recognize that health care is complex with personal, social, economic, and political factors that can be addressed independently or collectively. When you agree to represent others, listen to their stories to understand and then be a worthy messenger. Some of the characteristics you will need are flexibility, persistence, patience, and perseverance. Clearly articulate the reasons you seek to defeat the proposed legislation when you have the opportunity to speak with legislators.

Although you want to be consistent with your message, it is acceptable to use fresh approaches and different perspectives as you present your arguments. The vision for this kind of advocacy comes from your idealism and is fueled by passion for patients' welfare.

20. *Case:* **A patient is to be transferred from ICU to another nursing unit. He is afraid he will not get adequate care on the new unit. What can I tell him?**

There are four points you can make to help him have confidence that he is ready to move out of ICU. The first is to describe the transfer process. Let him know that you will give the nurses on the new unit all the information they will need to care for him. Next, explain that your intention in transferring him is to help him recover and to move him toward discharge by placing him in an environment that is more similar to his home. The third point is to describe the unit and the care he can expect. Schedules, increases in activity, and progressive self-care can all be discussed. The last point is to talk with him about the outcome of the hospitalization stressing the progress he has made thus far and reassuring him that this transition is the next step.

RESOURCES

Agency for Health Care Policy and Research (AHCPR). (1993). *Acute pain management in adults: Operative procedures*. Rockville, MD: Author.

American Nurses Association. (2001). *Code of ethics for nurses with interpretive statements*. Washington, DC: American Nurses Publishing.

American Pain Society. (1999). *Principles of analgesic use in the treatment of acute pain and cancer pain* (4th ed.). Skokie, IL: Author.

Chafey, K., Rhea, M., Shannon, A. M., & Spencer, S. (1998). Characterizations of advocacy by practicing nurses. *Journal of Professional Nursing, 14*(1), 43–52.

Greggs-McQuilkin, D. (2002). Nurses have the power to be advocates. *MedSurg Nursing, 11*(6), 265, 309.

Joint Commission on Accreditation of Healthcare Organizations. (2001). *Comprehensive hospital accreditation manual*. Oakbrook Terrace, IL: Author.

Luther, A. P. (2000). Advocacy—the cornerstone of professional nursing. *ORL-Head and Neck Nursing, 18*(4), 4–5.

Mallik, M. (1997). Advocacy in nursing—a review of the literature. *Journal of Advanced Nursing, 25*(1), 130–138.

McCaffery, M., & Pasero, C. (1999). *Pain: Clinical manual*. St. Louis: Mosby.

Studzinsky, S. R. (2002). Patient education trends [Electronic version]. *Advance for Nurse Practitioners, 10*(10). Retrieved from http://www.advancefornp.com

Chapter 3

Informed Consent: Ethical Issues

Susan B. Dickey

1. What is the difference between legal and ethical informed consent?

The idea of informed consent has its origins in law, ethics, and all healthcare disciplines, both ancient and modern, whereby a process must take place so that care rendered is a mutually agreed upon service between the provider and the patient. The legal idea of informed consent has its traditions in Anglo-American common law dating back to the 1700s. Legally protected interests in the United States include bodily integrity and individual autonomy. Both civil and criminal codes of assault and battery protect the idea of bodily integrity. Autonomy has its legal roots in common law, which was followed by the US Constitution.

The ethical basis for informed consent flows from classical Greece, where the promotion of autonomy and well-being were guiding principles. The ethical theory for informed consent emanates from two, sometimes competing, bases: deontological (rule-based) and teleological (right and duty in terms of good and that which produces good consequences) ethics. Ethical theory serves as "the rules behind the rules," whereas laws are more narrowly drawn from the ethical guidelines or normative customs of a society. Laws create specific protections; therefore, "informed consents" that are assumed by the individuals involved in the consent process to meet legal requirements may not satisfy the broader requirements for an ethically valid informed consent process. In many practice settings, a preponderance of obtained consents for surgery and other procedures fail to meet most ethically valid consent requirements; yet, neither patients nor providers may have an awareness or concern that a full disclosure process has not taken place.

2. How did the Doctrine of Informed Consent develop in the United States? What are other countries' approaches?

It is of historical interest to note that the issues in early, recorded cases were not concerned so much with self-determination, but with lack of information. Faden and Beauchamp (1986) discussed the four famous battery cases between 1905 and 1914 which formulated the basic features of the US doctrine of informed consent. The most important one was *Schloendorff v. Society of the New York Hospital* (1914), in which Justice Cardozo wrote "every human being of adult years and sound mind has a right to determine what shall be done with his own body" (p. 92).

The forces in the 1980s that further shaped the Doctrine of Informed Consent included the civil liberties revolution, the movement for consumer rights and advocacy, consumers who were better informed about treatments and the alternatives, and media coverage of medical issues. This media coverage included important mid-twentieth-century court cases about the shift from a professional to a patient-based standard of decision making such as in *Canterbury v. Spence* (1972). The *Canterbury* case was one of a series of cases tried in various levels of the courts that pushed to "permit patients to exercise choice concerning the risks to which they are willing to subject themselves" (p. 772).

Consent requirements in other countries follow the customs and the statutory laws or codes of their lands, unless they have developed their doctrines in Anglo-American tradition, which is based on case law. The US currently has the most scrupulous legal requirements for informed consent, since it houses a very litigious society.

3. What is the difference between informed consent for treatment *versus* informed consent for participation in research?

A scrupulous, higher standard of disclosure is always important for enrolling patients into research protocols. (See chapter 5 for standards of disclosure required for patients-subjects to participate in research.) Informed consent for treatment requires that a *process* occur between the provider and the patient (or legal guardians in the case of minors or the legally incompetent). It is not simply a matter of signing a consent form. The following transactions must have occurred in order for a valid process to have taken place:

- an explanation of the condition

- a fair explanation of the procedures to be used and the consequences

- a description of alternative treatments or procedures

- a description of the benefits to be expected

- an offer to answer the patient's inquiries

- freedom from coercion, unfair persuasions, and inducements

These criteria make up two of three components of a legally valid treatment decision: *voluntariness* and *information*. The third component is *competence*. The four tests of legal competency include:

1. evidence that a choice has been made

2. "reasonable" outcome of choice (the option the patient selects must correspond to the choice a "reasonable person" would make)

3. rational reasoning (the treatment preference was derived from rational or logical reasoning)

4. understanding (comprehension of the risks, benefits, and alternatives to treatment)

The idea of "understanding" is very complicated to measure, both in a clinical and especially in a research setting. *Legal competency* is not usually congruent with the construct of patient *capacity* (see question 5).

4. What are the important components for informed consent to treatment that a professional nurse should know?

Nurses have a long tradition and legal responsibility for patient education and emotional support during times of crisis or routine healthcare decision making. Therefore, it is natural for nurses to accept both legal and ethical responsibility for ensuring that patients are fully informed, regardless of the nursing role. You should know *all* of the important components of informed consent listed above in order to ethically fulfill your role as a professional nurse. Frequently, nurses give away their responsibility and role to people in other disciplines, such as social workers, for patient-provider interactions such as these.

5. How can I be sure a patient has "capacity" before obtaining informed consent?

(See chapter 13 on Long-Term Care for measuring *capacity*.) The idea of capacity encompasses an individual's innate potential for development and accomplishment. Inherent in this idea is that the person is able to use mental functions to learn, hold, and process knowledge. Capacity has both developmental components as well as mental status components. Examples of developmental components include school-aged children who are making the transition from the magical thinking styles of preschool to concrete reasoning, or becoming able to reason more and more abstractly as they move into adolescence.

Competence is a legal term, with the core notion defined as the ability to perform a task. The notion of variable competence to participate in the task at hand is a basic assumption in education, although not in health care. In health care, categories of persons such as minors, retarded persons, or the mentally ill are generally presumed incompetent to participate in healthcare decisions that relate to them. Competence is presumed in all adults unless they have been formally adjudicated incompetent. Interestingly, as long as adults concur with providers' recommendations (some of which are not in the best interest of the patient), there is no conflict. When providers consider patients' decisions not to be in their own best interest, questions about even adults' capacity and legal competence arise.

The assessment of competence in minors and adults with limited capacity is an evolving area of concern, especially when a parent or guardian is making a substituted judgment. These are the times when providers may seek intervention from the courts. The most important idea is that a full and thorough capacity assessment for the healthcare decision at hand has taken place, especially when the consequences of the decision to submit or abstain from treatment have life-transforming consequences.

6. How should informed consent be handled for the mentally ill who refuse treatment?

Posever and Chelmow (2001) proposed a process of *tripartite consent* for research in schizophrenia, which always requires a more exacting standard of disclosure than treatment, although ethically, it probably should not. This process calls for "oversight of consent by three professionals, each with a distinct domain of responsibility and expertise, and each with the authority to deny or accept a prospective subject's choice to participate in the proposed research" (p. 10). The question here is about treatment. In routine treatment, it is assumed that the provider prescribes in the patient's best interest. However, the team and family should be involved in order to secure the ethical participation of the patient in his/her care.

Carney, Neugroschl, Morrison, Marin, and Siu (2001) and Howe (2001) have developed and discussed a capacity assessment tool for people with variable competence, including the psychiatrically ill. They cite new scientific findings about the nature of decision making that are beyond the scope of this discussion, but suggest that those who show denial, exaggerate the tendency to see their problems as all or none decisions, or refuse lifesaving care may need shifting standards of competency.

7. How much knowledge and disclosure are needed to explain the percentages of risks, error, and benefits to be expected?

Knowledge and disclosure of the procedures or regimens to be administered should be in as much depth as the patients, including parents or guardians, are willing to tolerate. Rushton and Lynch (1992) suggested a strategy for involving people in their care by incorporating a family values history assessment. An offer to answer all questions should be made. In addition, the patient should be able to contact the provider involved in the consent process if there are additional questions or uncertainties.

If the provider feels at all uncomfortable that the patient is avoiding full disclosure, a family conference (with the patient's permission and participation) should take place. If family members' feedback is sought for legally competent patients, it must be with the patient's permission to remain within the ethical and legal boundaries of confidentiality and Health Insurance Portability and Accountability Act of 1996 (HIPAA). In the case of the mentally challenged or minors who do not meet the legal criteria for emancipation in the state where care is being rendered, opportunities should be provided not only for family conferences, but individual ones as well, so that all concerns may be expressed openly. This is costly and time-consuming, but will enable more autonomous participation in the future of the patient's health care.

The *provider-patient power differential* should always be considered when evaluating how much disclosure is necessary. Providers at work are usually in good health and often lack awareness of how much duress an illness imposes on a patient. Judgment in the otherwise competent individual may be challenged by the shock, disbelief, and denial of even minor deviations from health.

8. If a patient signs a consent form without reading it, is it legal?

Since signing a consent form has no bearing on whether a legal and/or ethical informed consent process has taken place, a signed consent form may be considered "legal." Providers must be able to document and demonstrate on recall that all attempts to ensure that a legally and ethically valid informed consent process has taken place. Literacy rates and language barriers are relevant here. Confidentiality may be severely violated when a family member is triangulated into a healthcare decision, especially a minor child, who is asked to translate, read, or explain about sensitive personal information, such as the disclosure of an HIV diagnosis or sexually related information. Legal requirements stipulate that a service is in place to ensure that translators of all languages are in place 24 hours a day. Most institutions meet this requirement with a telephone service, where the provider calls in to obtain a translator within a "reasonable" amount of time for a process of telephone consent. This may be awkward, but it's the best that some institutions may be able to accomplish in current times, given the many countries from which people immigrate to the US. Even large, urban university medical centers are having a great deal of difficulty and expense in meeting this legal and ethical requirement to ensure that a *valid informed consent process* has taken place.

9. What is the difference between an emancipated minor and a mature minor?

The answer to this question is based in legal, rather than ethical requirements. Most states have laws defining emancipation, whereas only a few have mature minor doctrines. Mature minors are defined as adolescents who have maturity in decision making and can participate in healthcare decisions.

Emancipated minors include those who are married and not subject to parental control. Pregnant or parent minors, college students, and military personnel are often included. The ethical nature of this question stems from the notion that "emancipated" minors are the ones who come to the attention of the healthcare system for problems that society considers to be troubled behavior; for example substance abuse, sexually transmitted diseases, or adolescent pregnancy. For the purposes of this chapter, an example of an emancipated minor statute from the Pennsylvania Code is included in Table 3.1.

10. Should parents be able to get information about emancipated minors' medical diagnoses?

This question becomes problematic when adolescents request that their healthcare information not be disclosed to parents (or legal guardians),

TABLE 3.1 Pennsylvania Law Regarding Consent by Minors: Prototype State Law for Adolescent Autonomous Decision Making

According to the following Pennsylvania Law, minors can give consent for medical care in the circumstances listed below: Pa. Stat. Ann. Tit. 35(1977 Bd. Vol.) (a) §10101; §10102; (c) §10103; (d) §10105; (e) Tit. 71, §1690.112 (1979–80 Cum Supp.).

The following individuals . . .	may give consent for . . .
A person who is 18 or older, who has graduated from high school, or who has been married or pregnant	medical, dental, and health services
A minor parent	medical treatment for his/her child
Any minor	examination or treatment for pregnancy, venereal disease, or any other reportable disease
A physician acting in good faith	may rely on the consent of a minor who professes to be one who is capable of consenting to care
A minor	diagnosis, care, and/or counseling for drug abuse. Physicians or organizations providing counseling to a minor may, but need not, inform the minor's legal guardian of care given or needed

especially if parents are responsible for paying the medical bills and refuse to provide insurance or other payment coverage without information. If the minor is legally emancipated in the state where care is rendered, then information is confidential and the provider has a legal and ethical mandate not to disclose it. It is the obligation of the provider or the "team" to meet with the patient, both separately and in a family conference, especially if parents remain insistent about obtaining information.

Nobody other than a parent or guardian in a bona fide legal relationship is entitled to information about a minor's healthcare status. This includes all other relatives, friends, and significant others. It is illegal for a minor to designate a healthcare proxy other than the legal parent or guardian under most circumstances, unless a court order is obtained and a *guardian ad litem* is appointed. The ethical approach to dealing with situations is to arrive at a consensus about which level of disclosure would make all parties involved the least uncomfortable, but to honor the request of the patient first.

11. Under what condition is it appropriate to obtain phone consent for anesthesia, surgery, or other procedures?

Phone consents are obtained frequently in the current healthcare climate, especially for children and other dependents (or "incompetents") with working guardians, for routine and emergency procedures. These conversations are often with a provider who will not be directly involved in the actual implementation. The conditions for a consent process include the following:

1. provider forges a relationship with the patient,

2. patient can re-contact provider with questions prior to or during a procedure.

Often, nurses or other hospital personnel are requested to "witness" such conversations by listening to the phone call on another extension, but in many cases phone consents are a two-way conversation between someone representing the healthcare service seeking consent and the patient or guardian. Professional nurses in all roles should approach these consent conversations with caution when asked to be a third party "listener," since they may be construed to be "in collusion" (have a conflict of interest) with the provider seeking consent.

12. *Case:* A wrong-site surgery has occurred on a patient. Do I, or does the physician, have the responsi-

bility to disclose it to the patient? What should I say to help the patient cope?

It is the physician's role to disclose the information. The nurse manager or supervisor should be notified. If satisfaction is not obtained this way, you may directly contact the risk manager of the institution.

If the patient or family member directly questions you about such an "occurrence," you will have to "think-on-your-feet" to answer without sounding off-putting. It is best to acknowledge that a problem has occurred; polite redirection of the conversation to the appropriate individuals is the most useful approach for all.

13. What is my ethical responsibility when I think the patient/family is being coerced or manipulated to sign an informed consent?

Coercion occurs when one person intentionally uses an actual threat of harm or force to influence another, such as the threat of abandonment. In cases of patient care, such threats can be so subtle as to go unnoticed, leaving the patient or significant others with only a vague sense of dread.

Manipulation represents attempts to influence that are neither coercion nor persuasion. Here the influence usually occurs with information manipulation—playing with data to change a person's understanding. This includes leaving professionally relevant information out of the consent process. Note that in the provision of "all the alternatives," there is no professional obligation to discuss treatments that do not fall within the scope of the healthcare provider's specific discipline, such as alternative and complementary supplementation. *Lack of full disclosure* is the most common form of informational manipulation. Therefore, due diligence by the nurse or primary care provider to see that full disclosure has occurred is of ethical importance.

Consent must be a situation in which there are no strings attached. If a patient refuses or is uncertain about a procedure or treatment that offers significant benefits, the clinician has the obligation to continue to inform and work with this patient and any significant others who may have a profound impact on the patient's thinking, including family members, legal guardians, or *guardians ad litem* (court appointed).

14. What is the "reasonable person" standard in informed consent?

The idea of the *reasonably prudent person* is a hypothetical construct that comes from tort law and is used by jurors *to develop and apply what they believe are community standards of reasonable conduct* (Fletcher, Lombardo, Marshall, & Miller, 1997, p. 93). This describes a patient-oriented standard, where the disclosure requirement is *as much information as a patient would want to know* (Fletcher et al., 1997, p. 93). If an average, reasonable person would decline to proceed with treatment in the face of fully disclosed risk, the physician who fails to make appropriate disclosure can be liable for any injuries that follow the treatment provided.

A landmark court case, *Canterbury v. Spence* (1972), changed the standard of disclosure from professional to patient based. The ruling concluded that if an "average, reasonable person" would decline to proceed with treatment in the face of fully disclosed risks, the physician who fails to make appropriate disclosures can be liable for any injuries.

The clinician's judgment about what to disclose is important, but that judgment should be based on his/her interaction with the patient and not on a predetermined script. This will help the clinician move to a patient-oriented standard of disclosure, as opposed to the earlier style of the mid-twentieth century, professionally based standard, in which "the degree of disclosure was primarily a question of medical judgment" (p. 772).

15. What are the exceptions to "requirement for informed consent" other than emergency?

Emergency is defined as when a patient is in a life-threatening situation and unable to consent. In this case, consent is presumed. Most patients who are of "danger to self or others," including suicidal patients, are presumed incompetent and unable to consent.

Other exceptions include incapacity, where the process must involve the surrogate decision maker, because the patient is unable to consent. Patient waiver, where the government waives the patient's or guardian's right to know, include national or state-level waivers. Examples include informed consent for vaccination programs and newborn genetic screening. However, today most states are careful to require consents for all immunizations, since the risk/harm ratio is not zero.

Another exception is therapeutic privilege, or the overriding of the patient's right to know by the provider, who determines that it is not in the patient's best interest for him/her to know information about diagnosis or prognosis, is another example of when the requirements of full disclosure have not been met. For example, a patient who is dealing with the final stages of congestive heart failure has little need to know he also has prostate cancer. This behavior stems from the ethical principles of beneficence or non-maleficence, in which the provider attempts to follow the dictum *primum non nocere*, or "do no harm" by leaving out information that may remove hope.

In addition, storage of tissue samples and their use for research or genetic products without the patient's knowledge are rapidly becoming issues of controversy when no consent process has taken place. Such devices for ignoring or obtaining consent should be evoked in only rare circumstances or when the risk for identification of an individual (as in research on an abandoned tissue sample) is extremely low.

16. What is the ethical grounding for informed consent?

The patient's right to self-governance or autonomy and in the principles of beneficence and non-maleficence is the ethical basis for informed consent. In tension with the principle of autonomy in informed consent is a traditional clinician-patient relationship in decision making in which the clinician makes the decision for the patient. This, when full disclosure requirements are not met, is a form of paternalism. In this professionally based standard, the assumption is that the patient is incapable of appropriate decision making. In the current climate, lack of full disclosure is not supported in the US by case law, and is, therefore, usually illegal. *Paternalism* is defined as the "interference with a person's freedom of choice or freedom of information," or the "deliberate dissemination of misinformation," therefore subjecting the patient to the clinician's judgment. The need for informed consent is an acknowledgment that provision of health care, or a medical procedure or act is meant to be done "for" and not "to" a person.

17. What does the ANA (2001) *Code of Ethics for Nurses* say about the nurse's role in informed consent?

Truth telling and the process of reaching informed choice underline the exercise of self-determination. Clients should be as fully involved as possible in the planning and implementation of their own health care. Clients have the moral right to determine what will be done to their own person; to be given accurate information and all the information necessary for making informed judgment; to be assisted with weighing the benefits and burdens of options in their treatment; to accept, refuse, or terminate treatment without coercion; and to be given necessary emotional support. In situations in which the client lacks capacity to make a decision, a surrogate decision maker must be designated, either by the patient prior to loss of capacity, by a family member, or by a court that will appoint a guardian ad litem.

18. *Case:* **A patient's parents are refusing treatment that could save their child's life. The physician and I have spent significant time providing information so that they can make an informed decision. What ethical responsibility do I now have, given that the parents continue to refuse treatment, not based upon religious convictions?**

You and, more importantly in this case, the attending physician should go through the entire chain of command. The administrator-on-call may seek a court order from a judge-on-call for just such emergencies. A court order from the judge may mandate lifesaving care for the child. In cases of religious beliefs, often much to the relief of the parents, this decision that goes against their religious beliefs is taken out of their hands. If the treatment to be rendered is to save the child's life, a judge may or may not order it, if it is considered "experimental" rather than routine care for the problem at hand.

19. Doesn't a patient have a right to know his/her diagnosis/prognosis?

In most instances in the US, cultural and sub-cultural customs have evolved such that the patient should be informed of his/her diagnosis and prognosis. In the case of sub-cultures where family members request that information be withheld, it is the ethical responsibility of the team to work with that family to try and move the family and the patient (if conscious and competent to the task at hand) to a point where the gravity of the situation is openly discussed. If after this action, it is clear that the patient is exercising the "right to not know," then the clinicians need to abide by the wishes of the patient. In situations where the patient is dying, the gravity of the patient's right to know is increased. Not knowing is depriving the dying individual of completing emotional tasks that may be of profound significance to both patient and family as life draws to a close. You are encouraged to read further in the topic area on end-of-life care, especially with regard to cultural competency. Suggested Web sites include: www.partnershipforcaring.org/statepolicy/audioseries/ or www.lastacts.org

Legally, informed consent is a requirement, unless there are extremely specific circumstances, especially if the person meets competency requirements and has reached the age of majority (over 18 years for most states). Informed consent is a trend even in pediatrics, although the information is tailored to the appropriate developmental level. Most children with terminal illnesses, even those as young as the age of 4 years, know when they are dying. Usually it is the parents who have trouble openly discussing such knowledge with a dying child.

20. **Case: A patient has a diagnosis of cancer of the thyroid with metastasis. As a nurse, what are my limitations in educating her about the odds of success with surgery?**

This is a question having to do with professional domain. Since the knowledge base required for answering such a question is usually held by general or otorhinolaryngologist surgeons, who would logically be the attending physicians, you are best off leaving specific questions of this nature to them.

There are circumstances where you may be functioning as part of that specific surgical service where you do have the knowledge base. However, this could become problematic at a later time if the patient claims that a medical decision was made about forgoing or proceeding with treatment based on a conversation with you, especially if it can be argued that the knowledge base is specifically within the medical domain.

RESOURCES

American Nurses Association. www.nursingworld.org

American Nurses Association. (2001). *Code of ethics for nurses with interpretive statements.* Washington, DC: American Nurses Publishing.

Berg, J. W., Appelbaum, P. S., Lidz, C. W., & Parker, L. S. (2001). *Informed consent—Legal theory and clinical practice* (2nd ed.). Oxford, UK: Oxford University Press.

Canterbury v. Spence, 464 F. 2d 772 (D.C. Cir. 1972).

Careny, M. T., Neugroschl, J., Morrison, R. S., Marin, D., & Siu, A. L. (2001). The development and piloting of a capacity assessment tool. *Journal of Clinical Ethics*, *12*(1), 17–23.

Committee on Publication Ethics. Topic: Informed Consent. www.publicationethics. org/uk/cases/zeroeightfour

Dickey, S. B., & Deatrick, J. A. (2000). Autonomy and decision making for health promotion in adolescence. *Pediatric Nursing*, *26*(6), 461–467.

Dickey, S. B., Kiefner, J., & Beidler, S. M. (2002). Consent and confidentiality issues among school-age children and adolescents. *Journal of School Nursing*, *18*(3), 197–186.

Faden, R. R., & Beauchamp, T. L. (1986). *A history and theory of informed consent*. New York: Oxford University Press.

Fletcher, J., Lombardo, P., Marshall, M., & Miller, F. (1997). *Introduction to clinical ethics*. Hagerstown, MD: University Publishing Group.

Howe, E. G. (2001). How to determine competency. *Journal of Clinical Ethics*, *12*(1), 3–16.

Nurses legal handbook. (2004). (5th ed.). Philadelphia, PA: Lippincott Williams & Wilkins.

Posever, T. A., & Chelmow, T. (2001). Informed consent for research in schizophrenia. *IRB: Ethics and Human Research*, *23*(1), 10–15.

Rushton, C. H., & Lynch, M. E. (1992). Dealing with advance directives for critically ill adolescents. *Critical Care Nursing*, *12*(5), 31–37.

Schloendorff v. Society of New York Hospital, 105 N.E. 92 (N.Y. 1914).

Steinke, E. (2004). Research ethics, informed consent, and participant recruitment. *Clinical Nurse Specialist: The Journal for Advanced Nursing Practice* (Vol. 18, No. 2). See continuing education program for this article, www.nursingcenter.com/ prodev/ce_article.asp?tid=494613 (Retrieved May 31, 2005).

U.S. Department of Health & Human Services. (2001). The Health Insurance Portability and Accountability Act of 1996 (HIPAA). http://www.hhs.gov/topics/ privacy.html

Chapter 4

Patients' Rights and Ethical Issues

Eileen Mieras Kohlenberg

1. What are the Patient Rights supported by the American Hospital Association?

The American Hospital Association (AHA) (1992), developed a Patient's Bill of Rights that includes 12 rights for patients and may serve as a model for establishing patient care guidelines. It is the Patient's Bill of Rights most often used in healthcare organizations. The rights include respectful care; current information about diagnosis, treatment and prognosis; informed consent; refusal of treatment; privacy and confidential communication; reasonable response to request for patient services; information about relationship of hospital with other institutions; information about research and experimentation; continuity of care; explanation of bill; and rules and regulations related to conduct of patients.

The nurse advocates for the rights of the patient in the following example. A child is admitted to a pediatric clinic with thrombocytopenia. Blood work and a bone marrow biopsy are conducted to determine if this condition is secondary to a diagnosis of leukemia. Two days later, the parents of the child voice concern that they do not have preliminary results of the tests. To protect the right of the parents and child to have current information about the diagnosis, the nurse immediately contacts the physician with the available results and asks the physician to contact the parents.

2. What are the Patient Rights supported by the American Civil Liberties Union?

The American Civil Liberties Union (ACLU) developed a Patient's Bill of Rights that identifies 23 rights for a patient (Springhouse Corporation, 2004). General categories include informed participation during care and research protocols; right to privacy regarding source of payment and patient information; right to accurate medical information regarding condition, care, and procedures; right to prompt attention; right to know professional status of caregivers; right to have access to an interpreter; right to access medical records and to receive a clear itemized bill for services; right to access consultant specialist; right to refuse treatments; right to access persons outside of the health facility; right to leave the facility and to have explanation for transfer to another facility; right to have notification of discharge 24 hours in advance; right to have counseling for financial assistance and timely notification of termination of third party payment; and 24-hour access to a patient rights advocate.

The nurse advocates for the rights of the patient in the following scenario. A patient enters the oncology clinic for radiation treatments that will occur over a 5-week period. A physician encourages the patient to take an experimental drug for anticipated diarrhea that may occur during the course of radiation treatments. The patient tells the nurse that she wants to satisfy the doctor's wishes, but is more concerned about the side effects of the experimental drug than the potential for diarrhea. The nurse informs the patient of her right to refuse treatment and documents the patient's decision in the chart.

3. A Patient's Bill of Rights that provides guiding principles for health plans sponsored by the Federal Government was approved in 1998. What are the patient's rights covered by this bill?

The Patient's Bill of Rights includes personal information disclosure; choice of providers and plans; access to emergency services; participation in treatment decisions; respect and nondiscrimination; confidentiality of health information; and a right to file complaints and appeals.

A patient on Medicare asks if his visit to the emergency room will be covered financially. The correct response is that federal health plans should provide emergency room payment for patients with acute symptoms of sufficient severity including severe pain that places that consumer's health in serious jeopardy, serious impairment to bodily functions, or serious dysfunction of any bodily organ or part. A patient advocate at the hospital or counselor in the cashier's office may answer questions.

4. What nursing guidelines may be used to uphold patient rights?

The National League for Nursing developed a Patient's Bill of Rights that may be used by nurses to uphold patient rights in the practice setting (Springhouse Corporation, 2004). Fifteen rights are delineated that include the right to accessible health care that meets standards of practice; courteous and nondiscriminatory health care; information about diagnosis, prognosis, and treatment; informed participation; qualifications of personnel providing care; refusal of observation by those not directly involved in care; privacy during treatment and during communication with persons of their choice; refusal of treatment; continuity of care; healthcare instruction; confidentiality and access to records; information regarding charges; and rights in the healthcare setting.

The following example illustrates the role of the nurse in upholding patient rights. An elderly man is admitted to the emergency room (ER) in respiratory distress. He is treated with inhalation therapy and given a prescription to be filled. He is discharged without further instructions by the physician. Before the patient leaves the ER, the nurse should clarify discharge instructions with the physician and instruct the patient using written instructions for the prescription, follow-up treatment, and future appointments.

5. The United States Senate has introduced a bill (S. 16) during the 109th Congress to reduce the cost of quality healthcare coverage and improve the availability of healthcare coverage for all Americans. What are the provisions of this bill that promote patient rights?

The purpose of this bill is to make prescription drugs more safe and affordable; to modernize the healthcare system with standardized measures of quality health care and data collection; to make health care more affordable for children and pregnant women and to reduce the healthcare costs for small employers. When this bill is passed, nurses will be in a position to advocate for these rights for their patients.

6. How does the Joint Commission on Accreditation of Healthcare Organizations (JCAHO) protect patient rights?

The Joint Commission (1987) requires that a list of patient rights be displayed in a prominent place in the healthcare institution and be given to each patient on admission. The list of patient rights varies among healthcare institutions, but generally addresses expectations set forth by JCAHO and federal legislation. The nurse should ask the patient on admission if he or she has questions or concerns related to individual rights as a patient. If concerns are identified, further consultation by the patient advocate in the hospital may be recommended.

7. How does the American Nurses Association (2001) *Code of Ethics for Nurses* protect patient rights?

The *Code of Ethics for Nurses* delineates nine roles for nurses. These include respect for the uniqueness of each individual; primary commitment to the patient and his/her rights; appropriate delegation of tasks for optimum care; continued personal and professional growth; improvement of health environments at national and international levels; advancement of the profession; and maintaining the integrity of the profession and shaping social policy. The *Code* provides guidelines for nurses to pursue in their careers. In the workplace, respect for the individual, commitment to patient rights, and appropriate delegation of care are expected. At a professional level, continued development is expected with contributions to the health environment, the profession, and social policy. These roles will help to maintain the rights of patients and improve health care.

8. *Case:* A patient questions items on a bill that has been received from the hospital for his care. What is the appropriate response?

The nurse should respond, "As a patient, you have the right to an itemized bill and explanation of expenditures. You may call the cashier's office or patient advocate in the hospital for assistance."

9. What patient rights are protected by the updated Health Information Portability and Accountability Act (HIPAA) in 2003?

The security of electronic-protected health information is addressed in the HIPAA update with implementation expected by health plans, healthcare clearinghouses, and certain healthcare providers. The act provides national standards for safeguards to protect the confidentiality, integrity, and availability of electronic protected health information.

If a patient asked if medical information was being shared with other pharmacies and health plans for marketing reasons, you could ensure the patient that the updates to HIPAA protect him/her from dissemination of patient information without his/her specific authorization.

10. What are the federal privacy standards to protect patients' medical records and other health information?

The federal privacy standards that were put in effect in April 2003 include provisions for access to medical records, notice of privacy practices, limits on use of personal medical information, prohibition of certain marketing practices, support of stronger state privacy laws, confidential communications, and a mechanism for filing complaints.

For instance, if the patient asked that the physician call him at work rather than at home to ensure confidential communications, this request should be honored under the new privacy rules.

11. *Case:* A competent adult patient would like to see his/her medical record. What should I do?

While the court system has determined that hospitals and physicians own the records of patients, the competent adult patient has a right to see his/her medical record. Hospitals and physicians may establish a procedure for access of medical records that must be followed by the patient. The nurse should advise the patient of the right to see his/her medical record and any procedures that must be followed.

A relative with the patient's approval, parents/guardian of a minor child, or parents/guardian of an incompetent patient may access the medical record under most circumstances.

12. *Case:* The patient would like to discuss his/her condition with a specialist consultant. What should I do?

The patient has the right to engage a specialist consultant. The nurse may suggest that the primary physician/healthcare provider be notified of the request. Conditions related to payment for a specialist consultant should be reviewed with the patient.

13. **Case: A competent adult patient refuses to take a medication. What are the nurse's responsibilities?**

The nurse should immediately stop preparations to administer the medication. The physician and nursing supervisor should be notified immediately. All actions should be documented in the patient record. Administration of a medication to a competent patient against his/her will constitutes battery.

14. **Under what conditions may a nurse administer a medication against a patient's will?**

Justification for administering a medication against a patient's will may include incompetence of the patient, protecting the life of the patient, and when refusal endangers the public. In these circumstances, the nursing supervisor and physician should be contacted to authorize administration of the medication. In some circumstances, a court order may be needed to proceed with the administration.

The following scenario provides an example of the nurse's role in this type of situation. An elderly woman with Alzheimer's disease is admitted with pneumonia to the Emergency Room. She is confused and refuses intravenous antibiotics. The patient's daughter who has durable power of attorney for healthcare decisions agrees that her mother should have the antibiotics. As the nurse, you contact your supervisor and the attending physician to further evaluate the situation. Since the patient is incompetent and the medication will protect her life, authorization is given to administer the medication against the patient's will. You document all actions in the patient's chart.

15. **Case: An adult patient has been asked to sign a surgical permit with language that he does not understand. What are the nurse's responsibilities?**

The adult patient should be advised to sign the surgical permit only if he has full understanding of the language. The physician should be contacted to further explain the language in the surgical permit.

16. **Case: A patient does not speak English and is only responding to questions on the admission interview by nodding her head. What should I do?**

An interpreter should be called immediately to translate for the patient. Only in emergency situations should treatment proceed without the availability of an interpreter. A list of qualified interpreters should be posted in the admissions department for use by all non-English-speaking patients. These interpreters should be educated regarding common healthcare terminology. Your responsibility as a nurse is to ensure that the patient has an interpreter available and that this person can accurately communicate regarding the patient's needs and care.

17. *Case:* **A patient desires to leave the healthcare facility without consent of the physician. What are the nurse's responsibilities?**

A competent patient has the legal right to leave the healthcare facility without consent of the physician. The physician should be notified, and the appropriate forms for leaving against medical advice (AMA) should be completed. If the patient refuses to sign these forms, documentation should be noted in the patient record. Appropriate discharge planning should be given to the patient.

18. **What do I do if an incompetent or dangerous patient desires to leave the healthcare facility without the consent of the physician?**

Patients who pose threats to themselves or others may be legally detained. Restraints, when necessary, may be used for psychiatric patients, prisoners, and violent patients. Call security for assistance when necessary and consult the hospital policies for specific interventions.

19. *Case:* **A competent adult patient with a Christian Scientist background refuses treatment in the emergency room. What should be my response to this patient?**

The nurse should respond, "As a competent adult patient, you have the right to refuse treatment in the emergency room. I am responsible for protecting your right to refuse treatment."

RESOURCES

American Hospital Association. (1992). A patient's bill of rights. http://www. hospitalconnect.com/aha/about/pbillofrights.html

American Nurses Association. (2001). *Code of Ethics for nurses with interpretive statements*. Washington, DC: American Nurses Publishing.

Guido, G. W. (2001). *Legal and ethical issues in nursing* (3rd ed). Upper Saddle River, NJ: Prentice Hall.

Joint Commission on Accreditation of Healthcare Organizations. (1987). *JCAHO standards*. Oakbrook Terrace, IL: JCAHO.

O'Keefe, M. E. (2001). *Nursing practice and the law*. Philadelphia: F. A. Davis Publishing.

Springhouse Corporation. (2004). *Nurse's legal handbook* (5th ed.). Philadelphia: Lippincott, Williams & Wilkins.

United States Senate. (2005). Affordable Health Care Act. http://www.theorator. com/bills109/s16.html

Chapter 5

Research in Human Subjects: Ethical Issues

Rose H. Mueller and Cindy Stern

1. What are clinical trials?

A clinical trial is a research study in human volunteers (human research subjects) to answer a specific health question. Carefully conducted clinical trials are the fastest and safest way to find treatments that work in humans. Treatment trials determine whether experimental drugs or new ways of using known therapies are safe and effective under controlled conditions. Prior to the implementation of a clinical trial, the treatment being studied must undergo pre-clinical testing in laboratory and animal models in order to determine biologic activity and safety. Once a new treatment has been tested in the laboratory, the Food and Drug Administration (FDA) must give permission for testing in human beings.

There are four phases of clinical trials. Phase I trials, the initial phase of human testing, are conducted in order to determine the safety and dose of the investigational drug. Phase II trials evaluate the effectiveness of an investigational drug for a specific disease or condition. In addition, the drug toxicities continue to be assessed. Phase III trials confirm study drug effectiveness, monitor toxicities, and compare the investigational drug to standard therapy. Phase IV trials are conducted after the drug has received FDA approval for marketing and continue to assess for long-term toxicities.

2. Is there anything I need to do before I administer an experimental drug to a patient?

Experimental drugs or investigational treatments are only permitted to be administered to human subjects in the setting of a clinical trial that has been approved by the FDA. The description of a clinical trial including background information, study objectives, eligibility criteria, treatment instructions, toxicity descriptions, patient monitoring parameters, statistical analysis considerations, and data recording requirements is contained in a document referred to as protocol.

Prior to the conduct of a clinical trial, the protocol must be reviewed and approved by an institutional review board, which is designed to ensure that the welfare and rights of study participants are protected (see questions 3 and 9). The Principal Investigator (physician with overall responsibility for the conduct of the clinical trial) and/or his or her designee is responsible for obtaining the study participant's consent prior to initiation of any study-related activities.

Patients who participate in clinical trials must meet specific eligibility criteria before beginning any study-related activities. Eligibility criteria help assure that the correct group of patients is being studied and that patient safety is being safeguarded.

Nurses who administer investigational drugs should be familiar with clinical trials procedures. Nurses confirm that IRB approval has been obtained and that patient informed consent has been documented. Nurses also secure information related to the specific study drug including administration procedures and potential toxicities. Nurses monitor and assess patient responses to the study drug and record their findings in the medical record.

3. *Case:* A depressed patient was placed on a clinical trial where she was given a placebo. I thought it was wrong to withhold effective therapy. Is that correct?

Research design comparing placebo versus treatment has long been controversial because of potential ethical implications. When a placebo is used in addition to standard therapy, there is little concern. However, when placebo is used in place of available standard therapy, questions arise concerning patients receiving less than standard care. Key questions to answer include the following:

1. What is the standard of treatment?
2. What is the purpose of the proposed research?

3. What are the risks to the participant who receives only placebo?

4. In assessing the risk of placebo to the participant, are the risks minimal and reversible or greater and/or irreversible?

The institutional review board (IRB) must consider the welfare of the individual participant as well as the welfare of those in the future who may benefit from the proposed research. When the standard of care is no therapy or observation alone, the use of placebo is less problematic. The informed consent must clearly explain the treatment regime, with or without placebo. It is wrong to withhold standard therapy in most cases, but the investigator must explain to the arena where the research is being conducted that there is sound methodology and minimal risk when using placebo instead of proven therapy.

Is it in the best interest of this patient to participate in a study that offers placebo or is it advisable for this patient to receive standard care? In the example of the patient above, the investigator must take into consideration the welfare of the depressed patient and weigh patient participation with the identified potential risks and benefits.

4. *Case:* **A patient was asked to participate in a clinical trial that compared a conventional treatment with a newer experimental one. Is it possible for researchers to choose ethically which patients get the opportunity to receive the newer treatment?**

When a clinical trial compares a conventional treatment (referred to as the control arm) to an experimental treatment (referred to as the investigational arm) neither the researcher nor the patient have the opportunity to choose which treatment the patient will receive. In order to eliminate the potential for bias, patients are assigned to treatment arms through the process of randomization, which is very much like "flipping a coin." When randomization is used, patients have an equal chance of receiving either the experimental or the conventional treatment. Treatment assignment through randomization is explained to the patient by the researcher or the clinical trial coordinator during the informed consent process.

5. Why are some patients offered the opportunity to participate in a clinical trial while others are not?

All clinical trials include eligibility criteria, which outline specific requirements for patient inclusion and exclusion. In order to facilitate accurate analysis of clinical trial results, it is important that the participants have similar characteristics that fall within the established criteria. For example, a clinical trial for lung cancer may be limited to patients with a very specific type of lung cancer such as early stage adenocarcinoma of the lung. Patients with advanced lung cancer or patients with squamous cell lung cancer would not meet the eligibility criteria and, thus, not be offered the opportunity to participate in the trial. The researcher and the clinical trial coordinator are able to identify which patients meet clinical trial eligibility criteria.

6. Is it unethical for a physician to receive financial reimbursement for enrolling patients in clinical trials?

Most clinical trials include financial reimbursement to physicians for patient enrollment. Concerns about potential conflict of interest may be cited because it has been suggested that physicians are enticed to enroll patients in those trials that offer financial reimbursement. Financial reimbursement is provided to cover the clinical, administrative, and data management costs that are incurred during clinical trial participation. Clinical costs can include examinations, procedures, or diagnostic tests that are required by the clinical trial. Administrative costs may include institutional review board (IRB) submission preparation and review, sponsor and patient correspondence, and drug inventory maintenance. Data management costs include the cost of hiring the personnel to perform data collection and submission. In addition, the data manager follows patient progress and monitors adherence to the clinical trial requirements.

If physicians have financial interests in companies or organizations that extend beyond standard reimbursement for enrollment, they are required to identify those interests at the time of informed consent. Physicians are guided by the ethical principles of beneficence (promoting the good for others), non-maleficence (obligation to do no harm), and respect for others (recognition of autonomy) in recommending clinical trials and in identifying situations that pose conflicts of interest.

7. *Case:* After 3 weeks of participation in a clinical trial, a patient wants to discontinue receiving the investiga-

tional treatment and switch back to standard treatment. Since she already signed consent, is she permitted to discontinue investigational treatment?

Clinical trial participation is always voluntary. Patients are permitted to discontinue participation at any time without negative effect on further treatment. As long as standard treatment is available and in the best interest of patient safety, this option should be possible. The informed consent process should include a review of the voluntary nature of clinical trial participation.

8. What are the ethical considerations for paying participants in clinical trials?

In some instances, participants in clinical trials are paid for their involvement. However, payment must be within reason. Excessive payment is considered coercive and not ethical. Therefore, most often payment is reflective of the costs of transportation, parking, or the time patients expend for assessments and follow-up.

9. What safeguards are in place to protect the ethical rights of clinical trial participants?

The Federal Government through the Food and Drug Administration (FDA) requires that every organization conducting human subjects research bring together an IRB. The IRB reviews each study and associated documents in order to ensure that the welfare of participants is protected. The Code of Federal Regulations guides IRB makeup and review. An IRB has the authority to approve, require modification in, or disapprove research.

Some of the specific areas of review include the following:

- **Review of Risk/Benefit Analysis.** One of the major responsibilities of the IRB is to assess the risks and benefits to participants in the proposed research. This includes identifying potential benefits of the research, determining the risks are reasonable, assuring that potential subjects will be provided with an accurate description of risks, and potential benefits.

- **Review of Informed Consent Process.** This ensures that potential research subjects are provided with an accurate and fair description of what the research entails, the risks/benefits, and assurance that participation is voluntary. All of the following must be clearly stated in the consent:

1. who obtains consent,

2. how to withdraw from the study,

3. any payment for participation or injury,

4. who to contact if the subject is injured or his/her rights as a participant are violated.

- **Selection of Subjects.** The IRB has the responsibility to ensure that the rights of a potential participant are protected in the recruitment of subjects and that subjects are not coerced in any way.

- **Privacy and Confidentiality.** The IRB ensures that the informed consent clearly states who has access to the participant's research records. This is separate from HIPAA authorization forms, which are signed prior to determining a participant's eligibility for the study.

- **Monitoring and Observation.** How the research will be monitored is part of the IRB review. The IRB has the responsibility to monitor adverse events (toxicities) that are reported during the course of the study. It is the investigator's responsibility in conducting research to report any adverse events immediately to the sponsor and to the IRB. The IRB has the right to observe the consent process in its quality monitoring process.

- **Additional Safeguards Such as Data Monitoring.** To be consistent, many cooperative research groups have independent data monitoring safety committees that report to the investigator and the IRB periodically during the research study. FDA requires reporting of any adverse events related to drug or medical device research studies.

- **Incentives for Participation.** Incentives may be paid to participants within reason. The IRB must determine that incentives paid to participants or investigators are not coercive. Any financial conflict of interest on the part of the investigator must be disclosed prior to IRB review.

- **Continuing Review.** Research protocols must have IRB review at least annually until the study is closed and all data collection has been completed. The IRB has the authority to request a more frequent review of an individual protocol. Continuing reviews are done in order to monitor the conduct of the research including number of enrolled patients, changes in the original study, and development of any adverse events.

10. What is a protected population?

Protected populations are considered to be at potential increased risk for undue burdens because of participation in human subjects research. These individuals are seen as dependent or as having compromised capacity for providing consent. Vulnerable populations include prisoners, economically disadvantaged, racial minorities, children, fetuses, pregnant women, and terminally ill individuals. The Code of Federal Regulations outlines specific protections for prisoners, fetuses, children, and pregnant women.

11. Who is permitted to have access to patients' medical records if they take part in a clinical trial?

Individuals or organizations that are part of the clinical trial and data monitoring process are generally permitted access to the patients' medical records if they take part in a clinical trial. These individuals may include the researcher or principal investigator, clinical trial coordinator, or other data management personnel and designated institutional review board staff. Organizations can include the clinical trial sponsor, the FDA and specific branches of the National Institutes of Health (NIH) such as the National Cancer Institute (NCI). The informed consent process should include a review of potential individuals or organizations that may have access to patients' medical records that pertain to clinical trial participation.

12. *Case:* A patient is considering entering a treatment trial, and as part of the study he is being asked to consent to blood/tissue banking for future research. Is this an ethical request?

Improved technologies are resulting in a growing interest in the secondary use of stored blood and tissue samples (tissue banking). The samples obtained at the time of diagnosis and treatment can be retained for an extended time and later used to answer research questions that had not been anticipated. Genetic analysis is the most common type of research done using stored materials. Several ethical concerns have been associated with this practice.

Collection and storage of blood and tissue samples for future research is not ethical unless full consent is obtained. Patients should be given the opportunity to refuse participation or identify limitations for the use of their samples and be recontacted for separate informed consent as each new project is undertaken, especially when the samples are identifiable and linked to the original donor. Researchers have been permitted to take already existing samples and make them anonymous for use in research without seeking consent, though this practice raises ethical concerns when the researcher had an opportunity to get consent, but failed to do so. Making samples anonymous and destroying any potential identifiers is helpful when the patient withdraws from the original study or has died.

Patients and families are advised whether the results of future genetic analysis will be provided. If this type of information is communicated to patients and families, the appropriate resources for confidentiality, education, support, and treatment, if available, should be provided.

13. **Case: A patient signed an informed consent for a treatment trial and she is to begin treatment on my shift. She says that she does not understand what it is all about, but signed the consent in hopes it will help her. What should I do?**

A patient's signature on the informed consent does not necessarily mean that the patient truly understands the purpose or procedures that are part of the clinical trial. Patients often agree to trial participation for various reasons including the hope that they will benefit from the investigational treatment. The researcher (investigator) or clinical trial coordinator should be notified if a patient does not understand the trial or procedures. Treatment should be withheld until the patient verbalizes a clearer understanding. The nurse should document the patient's comment and the subsequent actions taken.

14. **Case: I was present when a patient signed informed consent last week for a clinical trial examining an in-**

vestigational treatment for Alzheimer's disease. At that time, she was alert and oriented to person, place, and time. When I assessed her today prior to administration of the first dose of the investigational agent, she was confused and disoriented. What should I do?

A surrogate decision maker should be identified prior to the participant's consenting to the study in research involving participants with potential cognitive impairment, such as the patient with Alzheimer's. Federal law requires that a prospective research subject or the legally authorized representative provide consent to participate in a research project. The federal law defers to state law to define the legally authorized representative. Consult the investigator and/or the project coordinator to determine if this participant does have a legally authorized representative.

15. Is it unethical if institutional review board (IRB) members are paid?

The costs for IRB review can be significant in terms of time, materials, and record keeping. In many instances, affiliated healthcare organizations support the costs of having an IRB. Some IRBs institute fees for their services that support the cost of the operation. In addition, it is not uncommon for IRB members to receive financial compensation for their services.

However, the financial compensation is associated with the duties and not with the individual clinical trials. In addition, compensation for board members is on an equal basis.

16. *Case:* A patient's physician told him that his participation in a clinical trial was being terminated. The patient was very upset because he wants to continue receiving the investigational therapy. Is it ethical to terminate the patient's participation against his wishes?

When patient safety is of concern, the physician has an obligation to pursue an alternative course of care that will be in the best interest of the patient. Unacceptable toxicities in patients may warrant discontinuation of investigational therapy. Failure to benefit from a reasonable course of investigational therapy is another situation that may warrant discontinuation of that therapy. Termination of clinical trials occurs because analysis of data reveals that there is no significant benefit overall for patients. In some instances, there may be new findings or developments from other studies underway that lead to the termination of related projects. Finally, in some situations, the production of the investigational therapy ceases making the therapy no longer available for patient use. The informed consent process should include a discussion of the possibility of trial discontinuation.

17. Is advertising research studies ethical?

It is common to use mass media advertisement of clinical trial availability as a means of clinical trial recruitment. However, review of all forms of advertisement for recruitment by an IRB in order to assess that the content of the advertisement is accurate, truthful, and not in violation of an individual's ethical rights is necessary. In addition, the advertisements should not include any form of undue coercion.

18. Case: Staff in our office were told that if we recruit the most participants for a clinical trial, the researcher would bring us lunch. Is this coercion?

No, this is not coercion because there is no threat of harm, but it is persuasion. The ethical principles of beneficence, non-maleficence, and respect for persons guide nurses, as well as researchers. As long as these principles are adhered to, the benefit of "lunch" will not unduly coerce nursing practice and the recruitment of patients for clinical trials. It would only be seen as coercion if it propelled researchers to include participants who otherwise should not be included.

19. If there is a serious side effect while a patient is in a research study, do I report this to anyone other than the investigator?

Serious side effects should be documented in the patient's medical record and reported immediately to the investigator. However, in many situations when available, the clinical trial coordinator is initially notified and he/she in turn will notify the investigator. It is important to be aware of the procedure established for reporting serious side effects prior to administration of the investigational therapy. The clinical trial coordinator and/or the investigator are responsible for establishing and communicating this procedure. The investigator has the responsibility to ensure reporting of serious side effects to the institutional review board, the study sponsor, and in some cases, the FDA.

20. *Case:* **We have extra blood samples on hand for many of the patients. My colleague who is conducting a different study needs blood samples. Can I give her these extra samples?**

    If the blood was collected prior to the start of the research project, research can be done on those samples, if the patients' information is recorded by the investigator in such a manner that subjects cannot be identified. However, whenever possible, patient consent for use of blood and tissue samples should be obtained. On an increasing basis, clinical trials are including provisions for tissue and blood "banking" for future use in research. In these types of trials, consent for blood and tissue banking is obtained at the initiation of study participation. Patients are permitted to refuse to participate in blood and tissue banking and can withdraw consent at any time, once the original consent has been obtained.

21. *Case:* **The institution is participating in a clinical trial investigating strategies to prevent breast cancer and I have been asked to target minorities. Is it ethical to target minority patients for participation?**

    A review of clinical trials prior to recent years demonstrates that women and minorities are greatly under-represented. Although there are many reasons for this, knowledge about gender and race-related differences in drug safety and efficacy is quite limited. This is especially problematic when certain diseases are found to have higher morbidity and mortality rates in women and minorities.

    In 1986, NIH drafted its first policy promoting the inclusion of women in clinical trials. The NIH Revitalization Act in 1993 follows this policy and mandates the inclusion of women and minorities in all NIH-sponsored clinical trials.

Since that time many special programs and strategies have been implemented to increase the participation of women and minorities in clinical trials so that analysis of data can be applied to larger portions of the population.

22. Does the ANA *Code of Ethics* support nursing participation in clinical research?

The nine provisions of the ANA (2001) *Code of Ethics for Nurses* serve as a guide for nursing practice and support nursing participation in clinical research. The interpretive statement for provision number three specifically addresses the ethical considerations for nurses as they protect participants in research. It underscores the importance of the voluntary nature of patient participation in research as well as the necessity of informed consent and review by an appropriate IRB. In addition, the *Code* interpretive statements direct nurses to be cognizant of the protection of vulnerable groups such as children, prisoners, students, the elderly, and the poor. Finally, the *Code* recognizes the need for qualified individuals as the coordinators and directors of research.

RESOURCES

Amdur, R. J., & Bankert, E. A. (2002). *Institutional review board management and function.* Sudbury, MA: Jones and Bartlett Publishers.

American Nurses Association. (2001). *Code of ethics for nurses with interpretive statements.* Washington, DC: American Nurses Publishing.

Brody, H. (2002). What makes placebo-controlled trials unethical? *The American Journal of Bioethics, 2*(2), 3–9.

Cohen, P. (2002). Failure to conduct a placebo-controlled trial may be unethical. *The American Journal of Bioethics, 2*(2), 24.

Klimaszewski, A. D., Aikin, J. L., Bacon, M. A., DiStasio, S. A., Ehrenberger, H. E., & Ford, B. A. (Eds.). (2000). *Manual for clinical trials nursing.* Pittsburgh, PA: Oncology Nursing Press, Inc.

Penslar, R, & Porter, J. (2001, June). *Office for Human Research Protections IRB guidebook.* Available at http://www.ohrp@osophs.dhhs.gov

Veatch, R. (2002). Subject indifference and the justification of placebo-controlled trials. *The American Journal of Bioethics, 2*(2), 12–13.

Part 2

Ethical Issues at the Beginning of Life

Most of the controversial ethical questions occur at the beginning and at the end of life. In chapter 6, the issues of stem cell research, cloning, genetic testing, and other technologies are explored. Reproductive technology has enabled women an array of choices, but it rarely brings with it a moral consensus. Nurses working in NICU and Pediatrics will find the next chapters relevant to their everyday practice. Questions examine the benefits and burdens of treatment, setting boundaries with children and parents, and discipline issues. The questions and answers in part 2 challenge nurses to remember we are a pluralistic culture.

Chapter 6

Genetic Technology: The Frontiers of Nursing Ethics

Ellen Giarelli, Dale Halsey Lea, Shirley L. Jones, and Judith A. Lewis

1. What are a patient's medical options and legal or social responsibilities if he/she is at risk for a genetic disorder?

Genetic conditions may involve single genes, entire chromosomes or regions of chromosomes, or may be a result of gene-environment interactions. Genetic tests may be used to diagnose these conditions or identify people at risk for getting conditions later in life. As of this writing, there is no comprehensive law prohibiting discrimination on the basis of genetic information. There is also no hard evidence that such discrimination does exist, although anecdotes abound.

Patients at risk for genetic disorders may or may not wish to undergo genetic testing to quantify their risk. People have a right to information. They also have a right to not know this information. While one cannot mandate the sharing of the results of genetic testing among family members, genetic data often are shared among family members. This may result in an ethical dilemma for the nurse or patient who is faced with competing ethical obligations to safeguard the right to privacy for the patient, and also to safeguard the health of family members who may be unaware of their personal risk.

Most people believe that their privacy will be maintained if there is no insurance record of the tests being done, so they may choose to pay out-of-pocket for genetic testing. However, if life insurance or future health insurance questionnaires ask about knowledge of risk factors and the individual is not honest, then fraud may have been committed and the liability of the insurer may be limited. And, if the patient must receive health care for the genetic disease or to prevent the disease, then health insurance providers must be informed.

2. How do I explain genetic testing procedures and results to patients and capture the ethical issues?

Explain to the patient that *genetic testing* involves specific laboratory analysis of chromosomes, genes, or gene products (e.g., enzymes or proteins) to learn whether a genetic alteration related to a specific disease or condition is present in an individual. Genetic testing may be DNA-based, chromosomal, or biochemical. Genetic testing is usually performed on a blood sample. For prenatal diagnosis of a genetic condition, amniotic fluid or chorionic villi are used to gather fetal cells for analysis. In special circumstances, genetic testing is done using skin or other body tissues; for example, cells from the buccal mucosa or white blood cells. Genetic testing is beginning to be used to identify specific gene changes in a person that will help tailor treatment to that individual.

During counseling, the patient should be given the opportunity to talk about the ethical issues that may arise from using the technology. Table 6.1 lists the questions for ethical analysis. A good resource for learning more about genetic testing, the different types, and indications is the Gene Tests Web site at www.genetests.org

TABLE 6.1 Questions Applied to the Ethical Analysis of Issues Related to Genetic Testing

- What are the benefits and who will benefit?
- What are the potential harms and who will be harmed?
- What rights or responsibilities should be protected or adhered to?
- What relationships should be taken into consideration?
- Who should have access to the information generated?

3. How can I safeguard the privacy of a patient's genetic test results?

The ethical principles of beneficence, privacy, and confidentiality are relevant to this question. The protection of privacy is especially important for genetic test results because genetic information is not purely individual, but involves the lineage and ancestry of families. Genetic information may reveal the individual's health profile and the health profile of other family members, in particular the first-degree relatives (siblings, parents, and children). Some argue that because of the psychosocial risks associated with disclosure of genetic predisposition to diseases, genetic test results (and other genetic information) require special protection. Others argue that genetic test results should be protected in the same way as all medical information.

If the results of a genetic test are recorded in a patient's medical record, for example, researchers, insurance providers, healthcare professionals, and legal counselors among others may have access to this information. Nurses have an ethical and legal obligation to maintain the confidentiality of a patient's medical information including genetic information obtained in the context of health care. While nurses cannot guarantee privacy, they can take steps to ensure there is not a breach of confidentiality through carelessness or violations of federal laws, such as the Health Insurance Portability and Accountability Act (HIPAA). However, HIPAA provides explicitly that genetic information in the absence of a current diagnosis of illness shall not be considered a preexisting condition (for more information visit the Web site of the U.S. Department of Health and Human Services (http://www.os.dhhs.gov/ocr/hipaa). No comprehensive federal legislation has been passed relating to genetic discrimination in individual coverage or to genetic discrimination in the workplace. The existence and the provisions within laws to regulate discrimination varies across states.

4. Can a patient make an informed decision to "not be informed" as, for example, in Huntington's disease?

To understand the right to "not be informed," it helps to review the background of the process of informed decision making. If each component of informed decision making and consent is met, then the patient has the ability and information to decide to be informed or to not be informed of the outcome of the test, evaluation, intervention, or procedure (see Table 6.2).

TABLE 6.2 Information Requisite to the Process of Informed Decision Making and Consent

---

What is (are) the:

. . . purpose of the evaluation or test?

. . . pathophysiology and prognosis for the disorder of concern?

. . . rationale for testing or evaluation?

. . . benefit(s) of testing or evaluation?

. . . risk(s) of testing or evaluation?

. . . likelihood of a false-negative or false-positive result?

. . . alternative procedure(s) and intervention(s)?

. . . serendipitous and unexpected results that could occur?

. . . issues that will likely need to be addressed after testing or evaluation?

. . . implications of testing and evaluation for family members?

. . . counseling resources available to assist and support this process?

. . . confidentiality afforded the testing and evaluation process, including the findings?

For example, many individuals at risk for Huntington's disease (HD) choose not to have pre-symptomatic testing performed to determine if they have received the gene for HD from the parent with HD. Since this is a late-onset adult neurodegenerative disorder frequently without symptoms until after age 35–40, these individuals do not wish to know if they will or will not develop the symptoms of the disorder.

As a result, they approach reproductive decision making with the real possibility of transmission of the HD gene to the genetic child. (Note: If the parent has the HD gene, each pregnancy has a 50% chance of the HD gene being transmitted to the fetus.) For most this is not an acceptable risk. Thus, they are faced with a significant psychosocial dilemma: "Is it more important to not know my HD status or to prevent transmission of the HD gene to my future children?"

A novel approach through pre-implantation genetics diagnosis (PGD) provides the opportunity for at-risk individuals and their partners to have children free of the HD gene without knowledge of the HD status of the at-risk individual. To do this, the couple agrees after completion of the informed decision-making process to proceed with PGD without learning the HD status of the at-risk individual or any of the PGD embryos. This means that they agree to proceed with an intervention they may or may not require if the HD status of the at-risk individual were known. This decision to invoke "the right not to know" information requires that all facets of the informed decision making and consent processes be fulfilled prior to initiation of the intervention.

5. Does a carrier of a genetic disorder have the right to not inform his/her family of the possible risks for each of the members of that family?

The unique nature of genetic information creates an ethical quandary for individuals who have or are a carrier for a genetic disorder. Some individuals are compelled to share this information reasoning that every person wants and has the right to know so that he/she may also seek counsel and make his/her own life decisions. Still others recognize the dilemma of choosing to or not to share information with family members who also have the "right to know" and the "right not to know."

At present there is no legal requirement for dissemination of this information to family members. Moral expectations or judgments alone guide this decision. The nurse provides education and counsel for the individual to assist the person to understand and process the implications of each possible alternative decision. If the individual chooses to not share the information and withholding of that information has the potential for significant personal harm for another individual, then the nurse guided by the ANA (2001) *Code of Ethics for Nurses* is compelled to seek the assistance and counsel of the Ethics Board within the institution. The nurse does not have the legal authority to breach the confidentiality of the client-nurse relationship to disclose genetic information about one individual to another individual.

An individual is required to share genetic information about himself/herself when seeking health, disability, or life insurance. Should the individual choose not to do this, he/she has fraudulently provided information to the insurer and is at risk for reduction or elimination of benefits. An area not yet fully addressed by the legal system is the necessity or failure to disclose genetic information about oneself that predisposes the individual to adverse effects on his/her health and well-being when functioning in a specific work environment.

6. If I know a patient has a genetic disease that is inherited, but the patient does not want his/her family members to know, what should I do?

When a patient refuses to notify relatives who are at risk for carrying the same gene mutation, an ethical dilemma arises for the nurse who is faced with conflicting ethical obligations. On the one hand, nurses are obligated to respect and protect the patient's right to privacy and to maintain confidentiality. In doing so, they limit the dissemination of medical information to abide by the patient's wishes. On the other hand, nurses are obligated to prevent harm and promote the welfare of others. This suggests a responsibility to breach patient confidentiality and warn at-risk family members. Published guidelines are available to assist nurses when confronted with such issues. According to the *Code,* "Duties of confidentiality, however, are not absolute and may need to be modified in order to protect the patient, other innocent parties, and in circumstances of mandatory disclosure for public health reasons" (American Nurses Association, 2001). When a patient refuses to disclose information about an inherited disease or trait for which other family members are at risk, and for which there is prevention or medically accepted standards that will reduce genetic risk, then the nurse should collaborate with the healthcare team to encourage disclosure.

According to the American Society of Human Genetics the nurse and team are obliged to inform the patient about the implications of his/her genetic test results and about the potential risks to his/her family member. If the patient continues to refuse, then the nurse and healthcare team should seek ethical and legal support within the institution to help resolve the ethical dilemma.

7. Case: A patient's spouse is not the father of the unborn child. Do I have to reveal this if the patient wants genetic testing?

If the patient shares this with you in confidence, there is no obligation to reveal it, as your primary duty is to the patient. The patient should be aware that genetic tests may uncover the nonpaternity. In the pre-test counseling, you should include what results will be shared as the result of the genetic testing. For example, you may agree to share results about this particular fetus, including risks of recurrence based on maternity and fetal condition alone.

Part of the counseling should include information about the dangers of keeping family secrets, and the fact that information such as this often comes to light at less-than-optimal times. The patient may want to rethink her decision to not disclose the mispaternity. If her partner/spouse is unaware of the situation, it may be that the issue of mispaternity is an error, and genetic testing may relieve the patient of this anxiety if, in fact, her husband does end up being the baby's father.

8. Does a patient have to have a prenatal test if she does not want one?

It is important to understand that prenatal testing is performed to identify fetuses at risk for a genetic disorder and to identify fetuses at risk for poor perinatal outcomes. The key difference is the former usually does not have a therapeutic intervention available to favorably alter the outcome, while the latter testing is done because there is an appropriate therapy that can positively influence fetal/infant health and well-being. This is an important distinction given it has long been held that the mother has the right to choose or not choose to have prenatal genetic testing performed on the fetus. The legal system has upheld the sole right of the woman to choose the outcome of the pregnancy. For most genetic disorders identified through prenatal diagnosis, the mother and her partner are faced with the choice of continuing or not continuing the pregnancy; and if continued, raising or giving for adoption a child with minor to severe adverse effects on growth and development.

Conversely, the courts have intervened and mandated prenatal testing and therapy when it is demonstrated that the health and well-being of the fetus will be adversely affected by the mother's refusal of these procedures. For example, a healthcare provider may determine that an ultrasound (a noninvasive prenatal test) is warranted if by manual exam the uterus is found to be small for gestational dates. The sonogram evaluation may identify a pregnancy with diminished amniotic fluid that is the result of a fetal urinary tract outflow obstruction. This can result in permanent renal damage. In utero therapy is available to alter this outcome. Thus, the court may mandate the performance of the exam and subsequent intervention therapy holding that the rights of the fetus supersede the rights of the mother.

9. Is informed consent required before newborn screening tests are performed?

All states perform routine newborn screening. The type and number of conditions included in the screening panel vary from state to state. Many new parents are completely unaware that the newborn is being screened, what conditions are being screened for, and that the newborn screening tests are, in fact, genetic in nature. Most states have provisions so that parents can refuse to have the newborn screened, but this right of refusal is not always shared with the parent. The testing is covered under the routine admission consent in most hospitals. The principle at work is that knowledge is good, whether or not the parents wish to have this knowledge. The state believes it is acting in the best interest of the child and in the interest of the health of the public.

Parents have a right to know what the child is being tested for, what types of samples are taken, and what happens to any sample that remains after tests are performed. They have the right to know whether they can refuse testing. They also have the right to ask to whom the information will be given.

10. What disorders may be identified through an amniocentesis? What are the options available to a patient if a disorder is identified?

A variety of conditions can be identified through amniocentesis, including single gene disorders such as cystic fibrosis, chromosomal abnormalities such as Trisomy 21, and biochemical or metabolic disorders such as Tay-Sachs disease. Because of the increased incidence of chromosomal abnormalities in women over 35, the standard of practice is to offer prenatal diagnosis (e.g., amniocentesis) to all women who will be 35 or older at the time of delivery.

Specific indications for prenatal diagnosis using invasive means such as chorionic villus sampling or amniocentesis include advanced maternal age, having delivered a previous child with a *de novo* chromosomal abnormality, the presence of structural chromosomal abnormality in either parent, a family history of a genetic disorder that may be diagnosed by biochemical or DNA analysis, risk of a neural tube defect, or follow-up testing for abnormal maternal serum screening. In addition, amniocentesis for gender determination may be done if there is a family history of an X-linked disorder for which there is no specific prenatal diagnostic test.

There are many reasons women and their partners elect prenatal diagnosis. One reason is to reduce anxiety and provide reassurance to couples who are at increased risk for a particular condition. Some couples at risk for having a child with a serious anomaly who would otherwise choose to remain childless may attempt pregnancy with the knowledge that prenatal diagnosis is available. For conditions that require special intervention at birth, couples who elect to continue affected pregnancies can make appropriate plans for the site of delivery, the presence of specialists, and the preparation of the home for postnatal management. For some conditions, prenatal diagnosis may allow for prenatal treatment of the affected fetus; thus, preventing irreversible damage before birth.

11. What is "wrongful birth" and "wrongful life"?

"Wrongful birth" and "wrongful life" are used to differentiate between the individual and the parents of the individual who seek restitution for perceived malpractice during the care of a parent who is at risk for the transmission of a genetic disorder. Initially, courts did not award damages stating that the law could not draw a conclusion regarding the monetary value of "no life" compared to "life in an impaired state." This philosophy was later amended to recognize that the individual not only existed, but also suffered. Therefore, the parents, or the individual, were entitled to restitution if malpractice resulted in the undesired birth or life of that individual. Table 6.3 presents the similarities and differences between "wrongful birth" and "wrongful life" to assist the nurse to understand these terms and the associated ethical, legal, and social implications.

12. What are the ethical, legal, and social issues that patients confront when they decide whether to continue a pregnancy found to have a fetus at risk for a genetic disorder?

No matter the prevailing ethical, legal, or social issues, parents of a fetus found to have or be at risk for a genetic disorder face a myriad of personal questions for which they attempt to seek answers (see Table 6.4).

For many the crux of the ethical question is: "When does life begin?" Is it at time of conception, viability, or birth? Depending on an individual's personal response to this question, interruption of a pregnancy may or may not be a viable alternative. For example, a couple may wish to terminate a pregnancy, but because they live within a community that voices opposition to this choice, the woman and her reproductive partner may choose not to terminate the pregnancy. In contrast, a woman and her partner may fear social discrimination if they choose not to interrupt a pregnancy found to have a genetic disorder when the majority of their friends and family would choose to do so.

The legal issues revolve around the timing of the identification of the genetic disorder in the fetus and the length of time the parents require to

TABLE 6.3 Summary of Questions Associated With the Concepts of Wrongful Birth and Wrongful Life

	Wrongful Birth	Wrongful Life
Who brings the suit?	Parent(s) of a child	Child
What is the premise?	Parents perceive the child was wrongfully born.	Individual perceives he/she was wrongfully brought into existence.
What is the applicable field of law?	Tort	Tort
Who is at risk for such a suit?	1. Provider who did not provide full and appropriate prenatal information. 2. Provider who failed to make an appropriate prenatal diagnosis. 3. Provider who failed to make an appropriate diagnosis in the parent or sibling of a child yielding incorrect assessment of future reproductive risk.	1. Provider who did not provide full and appropriate prenatal information. 2. Provider who failed to make an appropriate prenatal diagnosis. 3. Provider who failed to make an appropriate diagnosis in the parent or sibling of a child yielding incorrect assessment of future reproductive risk.
What must be proven?	1. Provider owed a duty to the parent(s) on behalf of the child to act in a specific manner. 2. Provider breached that duty. 3. Parents suffered a significant injury. 4. Parents' injury is the result of the provider's breach of duty.	1. Provider owed a duty to the parent(s) on behalf of the child to act in a specific manner. 2. Provider breached that duty. 3. Child suffered a significant injury. 4. Child's injury is the result of the provider's breach of duty.

TABLE 6.3 *(continued)*

	Wrongful Birth	Wrongful Life

What have the courts determined?	Providers have a responsibility to:
	1. be informed and current in their knowledge of:
	
	   • prenatal genetic tests
	   • carrier screening
	   • fetal teratogens
	   • genetic basis of disorders.
	2. disseminate information to prospective parents.
	3. prepare materials that address the sociocultural needs of the parents.
		Providers have a responsibility to:
		1. be informed and current in their knowledge of:
		
		   • prenatal genetic tests
		   • carrier screening
		   • fetal teratogens
		   • genetic basis of disorders.
		2. disseminate information to prospective parents on behalf of the child.
		3. prepare materials that address the sociocultural needs of the parents on behalf of the child.

What are the ethical issues?	1. Parents would have chosen to not conceive a pregnancy or would have interrupted a pregnancy if appropriate information had been provided. 2. Providers must assess their own beliefs and values to ensure provision of nondirective, nonjudgmental dissemination of information.	1. Child would not have been conceived or born with the identified injury if appropriate information had been provided. 2. Providers must assess their own beliefs and values to ensure provision of nondirective, nonjudgmental dissemination of information.
What are the social issues?	1. Disruption of the expected parent-child relationship. 2. Long-term human and financial resources necessary to address the special needs of the child. 3. Parental chronic sorrow and the associated sequela.	1. Quality of life for the child with a significant alteration in their health, well-being, and/or life expectancy. 2. Long-term human and financial resources necessary to address the special needs of the child. 3. Care of the child if their parents pre-decease them.

TABLE 6.4 Questions a Parent May Ask About a Fetus at Risk for a Genetic Disorder

What is the prognosis for the child?	Is there treatment or therapy available?
How can I love and care for a child with this genetic disorder?	What if my partner does not agree with my wishes for the pregnancy?
Should I continue the pregnancy and place the child for adoption after he/she is born?	Do I have the moral right to give birth to a child with a genetic disorder?
Can I willingly choose to voluntarily interrupt a pregnancy?	If I do, will my child agree with that decision as they grow older?
If I do, do I have the right to grieve the loss of my child?	How do I tell my family (or friends, or coworkers) I am no longer pregnant?
Who will care for my child when I die?	What and how much should I tell them about their condition?
Is it appropriate to expect my other children to care for this child when I can not?	What will they think of my decision?

make an informed choice about the continuation or interruption of the pregnancy. Voluntary interruption of a pregnancy during the first trimester of a pregnancy may be done for medical or social reasons. Second trimester termination of a pregnancy is legally permitted up to 24 weeks in the United States. However, there is very limited availability of this service; and the service will not be provided unless there is a therapeutic reason for the interruption of the pregnancy.

13. What are some of the ethical concerns associated with cloning and stem cell research?

Ethical issues that enter discussions about the morality of cloning may overlap those about stem cell research. The main ethical issue involving embryonic stem cell research focuses on the status of the human embryos. Some key ethical positions related to using human embryos in stem cell research are:

- **Position 1.** Embryos are human individuals and should not be used or destroyed for research purposes.

- **Position 2.** Embryos do not have the same status as a fetus or a baby and can be used for research.

- **Position 3.** Embryos should not be created for research, but can be used if they are left over from in vitro fertilization procedures.

- **Position 4.** Embryos are clusters of cells no different from other cells and can be created specifically for use in research.

Because research with adult stem cells is not as ethically problematic, research continues unabated in this area. The principle of equipoise or balance of risks to benefits (or fears to hopes, or negative to positive outcomes) is often cited in the ethical arguments for and against cloning. The principle fear is that the technology of cloning and stem cell research will be misused or abused. This fear can be placed in the historical context of the use of "genetic science" to achieve eugenic ends in the U.S. and in Europe in the early 1900s.

In addition, cloning is expensive and inefficient (90% of attempts fail), the offspring may be unhealthy and die young or mysteriously, and cloned animals have a higher rate of infection, tumor growth immune systems, and other disorders. The benefits of cloning are to repopulate endangered animals or those difficult to breed, and to develop and reproduce animals with special qualities that can be used to produce medicines, stem cells, and replacement body parts and organs. Cloned animals can be used as models for studying human disease and, therefore, can be instrumental in efforts to find cures. Physicians from the American Medical Association and scientists with the American Association for the Advancement of Science have issued formal public statements advising against reproductive cloning.

14. What are the potential benefits and risks to patients who participate in stem cell research?

For some, the use of stem cells from embryos and human fetuses is controversial; for others, such research holds great promise for alleviation of disease and suffering. Most patients receiving stem cell therapy have diseases of myeloid or lymphoid systems (e.g., aplastic anemia, severe combined immunodeficiency). They may also have dysfunctional disorders such as thalassemia or neoplastic disorders such as myelodysplasia, leukemia, or lymphoma. Stem cell treatment for these patients may be autologous (using their own stem cells), syngenic (identical twin donor), or most commonly from an allogenic donor (sibling or matched donor).

Complications from stem cell therapy mainly arise with allogenic stem cell therapy and include acute or chronic graft versus host disease. Other complications are related to the chemotherapy and radiation therapy prior to stem cell therapy; these include infectious complications, vascular, and hepatic complications. For some patients there are significant psychosocial consequences, such as feelings of guilt at needing to call on a sibling to be a stem cell donor, fear of treatment failure, depression from disease and treatment complications, and concerns regarding healthcare treatment costs. There have been recent reports that some children with Severe Combined Immunodeficiency disease who have undergone stem cell therapy have developed leukemia. Patients with Parkinson's disease are now participating in stem cell therapy research trials using human embryonic stem cell implantation. Side effects reported with Parkinson's disease have included severe and uncontrollable dyskinetic side effects after 1–3 years. Nurses can share with patients that although there is hope that stem cell research will improve the health and well-being of individuals, the long-term side effects of stem cell therapies are not completely understood.

15. Who has access to the stem cells found in umbilical cord blood if it is required for treatment (the person who donated it or the general public)?

Cord blood is not different from any other body part or body fluid in terms of ownership. When tissue is donated, it is appropriate for the donor, in this case the mother, to be informed about what will be done with the sample, how it will be used, and for the donor to provide consent. If there are any limitations to how the donor would like the sample to be used, then the donor has the right to list these at the time the sample is donated. If the sample is to be used for research, the consent form will have been approved by an institutional review board. If it is to be used for treatment, then the treatment facility is responsible for having the appropriate consent form. Once the sample is donated and the consent is signed, the donor must abide by the terms of the consent and this usually includes forfeiting the right to control the sample in the future. The public use sample is anonymous and is made available for research or patient care.

16. What are a person's rights after he/she donates stem cells?

This question raises two general ethical issues: (1) the ownership of biological samples and (2) the protection of an individual from harm. On the ownership of biologic samples, often stem cells are donated as part of a research protocol or for a special medical need of a patient whose disease may be treated with donated stem cells (e.g., bone marrow transplant for leukemia and the medical procedure to harvest stem cells). Typically, the consent will include a waiver of ownership or otherwise specify that upon the donation of cells the donor relinquishes all proprietary rights to the cells and beneficiary rights to the outcome of the use of the cells in research or medical practice. Once donated, all rights are transferred to the new "owner."

With regard to protection from harm, donors of stem cells have the same right to protection from harm during donation as during any medical procedure. In some uses, specimens are identifiable or capable of being linked to databases where identification is possible. This makes confidentiality a central concern. The donor retains the rights to have confidentiality and privacy protected by the removal of all identifying information from the bio-sample.

17.   What are the risks of gene therapy?

As with other new treatments for diseases, the ethical issue of most concern in somatic cell gene therapy is the principle of non-maleficence or "first do no harm." When discussing the option to participate in an experimental trial using gene therapy, the patient must be informed of all the risks. At the present level of technology there are many significant risks and few benefits to this novel therapy. The risks are listed in Table 6.5.

In germ-line gene therapy the ethical debate confronts the distinction between using a technology to cure versus using one to enhance. There is

TABLE 6.5   Risks of Gene Therapy

Risk	Source
Problems with viral and bacterial vectors	Viral vectors may introduce a disease, toxicity, inflammatory responses. They may not be effective.
Immune response	Foreign objects introduced into human tissues may cause immune response that is mild to severe (anaphylaxis).
Unanticipated negative consequences	Technology is too new to specify.

little argument against using a technology to cure deadly or crippling diseases. Also, there is less concern for the use of a technology that can pinpoint a defective gene in a germ-line cell, replace it with a normal version, and effectively prevent disease. Some of the diseases that potentially could be detected and prevented before birth are Down syndrome, Hemophilia A, Huntington's disease, Tay-Sachs disease, and cystic fibrosis, as well as certain kinds of cancers or cancer syndromes caused by a single gene mutation.

18. What are the issues related to plant and animal genetic engineering?

Genetic modification (GM) is used to describe the genetic engineering of plants and animals, and is a special set of technologies that alter the genetic makeup of living organisms, such as animals, plants, or bacteria, and dates back to the 19th century. Combining genes from different organisms is known as recombinant DNA, and the resulting organism is said to be: "genetically modified," "genetically engineered," or "transgenic." GM products include medicines and vaccines, foods and food ingredients, animal feeds, and fibers. In 2000, about 109.2 million acres were planted with transgenic crops that were primarily engineered to be insect and weed resistant. These crops included cotton, corn, soybeans, virus-resistant sweet potato, rice with increased iron and vitamin A content, plants that can survive extremes of weather, low-caffeine coffee beans, and slow-softening tomatoes. In 2000, 99% of the global transgenic crops were produced in the United States, Argentina, Canada, and China. It is likely that your patients have consumed one of these GM foods or a product that combines GM grains with naturally occurring grains. However, foods or food products will only carry a GM label if the manufacturer chooses to include this information. GM labeling is not mandatory in the United States.

The ethical controversies deal with access to and fair distribution of resources, truth in advertising, and inability of the consumer to evaluate the balance of risks to benefits when the risks are largely unknown. Table 6.6 lists the potential benefits and risks of genetically modified products and Table 6.7 lists the ethical controversies that will continue to be debated.

19. How can I maintain competency in the provision of genetic health care?

Health professionals should know what the competencies are in the provision of genetic health care. The National Coalition for Health Professional Educa-

TABLE 6.6 Potential Benefits and Risks Genetically Modified Biologic Products Potential Benefits

Crops	Animals	Environment	Society
Enhanced taste and quality	Increased resistance	Bio-insecticides	More food for population
Reduced growing time	Increased productivity	Bio-herbicides	Solution to world hunger
Increased nutrients	Increased hardiness	Better waste management	Availability of medicines
Improved resistance	More meat, eggs, milk		
New products	Improved animal health		
New technologies			

Potential Safety Risks of GM Biologic Products

- Human health impact: allergens
- Human health impact: transfer of antibiotic resistance
- Human health impact: unknown
- Unknown environmental impact
- Unintended transfer of transgenes through cross-pollination, rise of super weeds
- Unknown effect on other organisms
- Loss of flora and fauna biodiversity
- Insect pests will evolve and develop tolerance to GM pesticides, rise of super bugs

tion in Genetics (NCHPEG) created a list of competencies for all healthcare professionals. This listing can be found at the Web site www.nchpeg.org. Once familiar with these, there are many genetics educational resources available for continuing education in genetics. NCHPEG has a listing of available genetics educational programs. Many are self-study CD-ROMs or Web-based programs for convenience and ease of use. The March of Dimes has a CD-ROM and Web-based program called *Genetics and Primary Care Practice* that is a useful resource for nurses and other health professionals. Professional groups such as the Oncology Nursing Society, the Association

TABLE 6.7 Ethical Controversies of Genetically Modified Crops

- Domination of world food production by a few companies
- Increasing dependence on industrialized nations by developing countries
- Tampering with nature by mixing genes among species
- Truth in advertising about sources of food products
- Mixing GM crops with non-GM crops
- Foreign exploitation of natural resources
- Violation of a natural organism's intrinsic values
- Stress for the organism; innocent creatures may be hurt

of Women's Health, and Obstetrical Neonatal Nursing have special interest groups and newsletters on genetics topics to keep their members informed and up to date. The International Society of Nurses in Genetics, Inc. (ISONG), the authority in genetic nursing, holds annual educational conferences that provide continuing educational credits for nurses in genetics. The ISONG Web site offers other listings and links to genetics educational offerings for nurses: www.isong.org

20. What are the required qualifications for nurses who do genetic counseling for couples?

A nurse who does counseling for couples who receive genetic health services is a licensed professional nurse with graduate level course work in genetics and who is either a board-certified genetic counselor or is an advanced practice nurse in genetics. These nurses perform risk assessments, analyze the genetic contribution to disease risk, and talk with patients and families about the impact of risk on healthcare management. They also provide education about genetic testing, provide nursing care to patients and families who have or who are at risk for genetic conditions, and conduct research in genetics.

Nurses specialize in genetics practice at both basic and advanced levels. Credentialing for genetics nurse specialists that recognizes these levels is available through the Genetics Nursing Credentialing Commission (GNCC), the authority on genetic nursing credentials (www.geneticnurse. org). Nurses who have a GCN are baccalaureate prepared, licensed, registered nurses who have received specialty credentialing as a Genetics Clinical Nurse (GCN). Nurses with advanced training—APNG—are licensed, registered nurses with a master's degree who have received specialty credentialing as an Advanced Practice Nurse in Genetics. The American Nurses Association has published a document on the *Scope and Standards of Genetics Clinical Nursing Practice* (1998) written by the International Society of Nurses in Genetics, Inc. This document provides a detailed description of roles and responsibilities of both the clinical nurse and the advanced practice nurse in genetics.

RESOURCES

American Nurses Association. (2001). *Code of ethics for nurses with interpretive statements—Provision 3: Confidentiality.* Retrieved from http://www.nursing world.org/ethics/Code/ethicscode150.htm#prov3

Buchanan, A., Brock, D. W., Daniels, N., & Wilker, D. (2000). *From chance to choice: Genetics and justice.* New York: Cambridge University Press.

Chapman, A. R., Frankel, M. S., & Garfinkel, M. S. (1999). *Stem cell research and applications: Monitoring the frontiers of biomedical research.* Newtown, MA: American Association for the Advancement of Science and the Institute for Civil Society.

Giarelli, E. (2003). Genetic testing and the threat to being: Toward a new bioethical ideal for genetic nursing care. *Nursing Ethics, 10*(3), 255–268.

Giarelli, E., & Jacobs, L. (2000). Issues related to the use of genetic material and information. *Oncology Nursing Forum, 27*(3), 459–467.

Human Genome Project. http://www.ornl.gov/TechResources/Human_Genome/ else/legislation.html

Jones, S. L. (2000). Reproductive genetic technologies: Exploring ethical and policy implications. *AWHONN Lifelines, 4*(5), 33–36.

Lea, D. H. (2003). Handling genetic information responsibly. In A. Tranin, A. Masny, & J. Jenkins (Eds.), *Genetics in oncology practice: Cancer risk assessment* (pp. 243–262). Pittsburgh, PA: Oncology Nursing Society.

Lea, D. H. (2002). Position statement: Integrating genetics competencies into baccalaureate and advanced nursing education. *Nursing Outlook, 50*(4), 167–168.

Lewis, J. A. (2003). Genetic testing: A personal story of one nurse's involvement in health policy. *Newborn and Infant Nursing Reviews, 3*(1), 11–12.

Lewis, J. A. (2001). The human genome and public policy: A nursing perspective. *Journal of Obstetric, Gynecologic and Neonatal Nursing, 30*(5), 541–545.

National Conference of State Legislatures. http://www.ncsl.programs/health/ Genetics/chhealthins.htm

The New York Times. http://www.nytimes.com/library/national/science/health/ gm-index.html

Nussbaum, R. L., McInnes, R. R., & Willard, H. F. (2001). Thompson & Thompson *Genetics in medicine* (6th ed.). Philadelphia: W. B. Saunders Company.

The Star Foundation. (2002). *Human stem cells: An ethical overview.* Minneapolis, MN: University of Minnesota's Center for Bioethics. http://www.bioethics.umn. edu

Chapter 7

Reproductive Technology: Ethical Issues

Mary English Worth

1. What are the primary ethical issues for couples wishing to pursue assisted reproductive technology (ART) for treatment of infertility?

There are many ethical concerns regarding the use of in vitro fertilization (IVF), which were first raised in the 1970s with the birth of Louise Brown, and continue to be debated today. Innovations in the application of IVF include the use of donor gametes; gestational carrier/surrogacy; cryopreservation of gametes, embryos, and male and female reproductive tissue; embryo biopsy for preimplantation genetic analysis; and intracytoplasmic sperm injection (ICSI) for severe male infertility. These advancements have added new dimensions and complexity for decision making by those seeking treatment. Couples may be forced to make decisions at a time when they are under a great deal of stress and are psychologically vulnerable. Their focus to achieve pregnancy may supersede their ability to consider fully the ramifications of treatment.

Ethical questions of individual harm and benefit to the patient, potential child, and society, as well as respect for autonomy are central to the ethical dilemmas posed to patients in their decision making. Possible ethical dilemmas include:

1. Personal comfort with a nontraditional form of achieving pregnancy.

2. Lingering controversy over using potent fertility drugs, which may increase chances of ovarian cancer and possibly other reproductive cancers.

3. Number of embryos to be replaced to maximize the chances of pregnancy, while minimizing the chances for a multiple pregnancy.

4. Risk of multiple pregnancies and, therefore, the potential for complications during pregnancy, delivery, and neonatal period. The concerns of prematurity and its possible detrimental effects on normal growth and development of infant.

5. Conflicted feelings regarding multi-fetal reduction.

6. Use of cryopreservation of any embryos not replaced in a given treatment cycle and the decision making regarding the ultimate disposition of any unused embryos.

7. Balancing realism with optimism for success while withstanding the physical, emotional, and financial drain on overall quality of life.

In addition, couples that choose to pursue IVF using a third party donor also must deal with the loss of at least one partner's genetic makeup. This asymmetry in biologic connection to the child may create conflicts. A major ethical question today is whether a child conceived from donor gametes has the right to know his/her origins for reasons of heredity and self-identity. Secrecy versus disclosure is an issue that requires deep exploration, which is best done before treatment begins. With the support and assistance from a mental health professional, the individual couple can discuss the potential impact their decision (to tell or not to tell) will have on them as individuals, as parents, and as a family.

2. What resources are available for patients wishing to pursue ART for the treatment of infertility?

The National Infertility Association, with its national network of over 50 chapters, was established in 1974. Its mission is (1) to provide timely compassionate support and information to people experiencing infertility and (2) increase public awareness of infertility issues through support, public education, and advocacy. The Web site features a breadth of publications and fact sheets covering the full scope of infertility diagnosis and treatment, as well as the physical, emotional, legal, and administrative aspects of infertility. Members can take full advantage of the full range of services on a national, as well as local, level including the helpline, support networks, educational programs, and online chat rooms.

The American Society for Reproductive Medicine (ASRM), the primary professional organization for practitioners in reproductive endocrinology and infertility, is an organization devoted to advancing knowledge and expertise in reproductive medicine and biology. In addition, the Society staffs an office in Washington, D.C., for its activity in legislative and patient advocacy efforts. The ASRM also has a strong commitment to patient education with a library of information available in print, as well as on the Web, addressing diagnostic and treatment options.

Both of these organizations provide links to specific, credible organizations that provide specific disease-related information or emotional support resources.

3. How do fertility clinics determine their success rates?

Ethical issues arise when clinics use reports describing their success rates to promote their programs, or use the results to compare their results with other programs. Full disclosure of how success rates and pregnancy outcome data are generated and the patient selection criteria used is an ethical obligation of all programs in the public arena, such as with the patient information seminars, or in any written information distributed to prospective patients.

Patients must be advised that these reports cannot be used for accurate comparison of programs. Some programs have careful selection criteria, only treating patients who have the highest chances for success, such as younger women. Others may have more open selection criteria, accepting those with reasonable chances for success, but for whom treatment may be more complicated.

The implementation of the 1992 Fertility Clinic Success Rates and Certification Act began in 1995 in an effort to provide consumer protection for those seeking treatment with assisted reproduction. The Society for Assisted Reproductive Technology (SART), an affiliated society within the ASRM, RESOLVE (NIA), and the Centers for Disease Control (CDC) work in concert to publish the annual *National Summary of Fertility Clinic Reports*, compiled from all clinics reporting data to SART. Since the single most important factor for success in a non-donor egg cycle is maternal age, cycle and outcome data are categorized by maternal age (< 33, 34–39, and > 40), as well as with/without a male factor. In addition, these organizations provide access, through their Web sites, to the clinic-specific reports, current and past.

4. Should there be age limits for egg donation recipients?

The application of IVF to enable infertile women refractory to treatment to pursue pregnancy has opened up the possibility of any woman with an intact uterus to pursue pregnancy with the use of donor eggs. A central ethical concern that continues to generate great debate in the ART community is the practice of this technology for postmenopausal women. The reality is that a limited number of postmenopausal women seek treatment with egg donation.

In fact, the population most seeking egg donation is women with premature ovarian failure and the peri-menopausal woman, who have failed IVF using her own eggs because of reduced ovarian reserve. These groups have spurred increased interest and growth in this option. Reported pregnancy rates of women over 39 using their own eggs range from 5 to 10% due to the naturally declining ovarian reserve. After exhaustive attempts and the emotional and financial drain of trying to conceive, these women can be treated much more efficaciously using egg donation, yielding success rates of 70 to 90% per treatment cycle. Most programs reported that they follow the ASRM recommended guidelines for treatment and have an age restriction, with an average range of 47–48 at time of treatment.

The ASRM Ethics Committee (2002) recommended limiting egg donation to women (egg recipients) who are within the limits of the normal reproductive life span. The recommendation by ASRM is based on medical, ethical, and social reasons. Pregnancy in the older woman is more likely to be complicated by increased cardiovascular risk, gestational diabetes, multiple gestation (inherent in IVF multiple embryo transfer), preterm labor, pre-eclampsia, and increased likelihood of an operative delivery.

The main ethical issue is whether serving this population of women is in the best interest of the mother, child, and family as a unit. Does the "older mother" have the capacity to endure the social and psychological stresses of parenting, especially with the increased risk of multiple gestation?

Social concerns primarily center on what is in the best interest and welfare of the child, as well as how he/she will socially adjust to the potential stigma of having older parents. Family and financial provisions and support systems need to be in place should his/her parent die or become physically or mentally incapacitated to care for the child prior to the child's reaching adulthood.

Despite continued debate and discussion within, there is a lack of consensus among physicians, ethicists, nurses, embryologists, and mental health professionals as to whether access to egg donation should be restricted. A few programs around the country are strong advocates for women having the right to pursue egg donation at any age, but also consider the aforementioned issues in patient evaluation and medical clearance.

It is the age of the egg not the uterus that precludes pregnancy in the woman of advanced maternal age. Pregnancies have been achieved and successfully delivered in postmenopausal women in their 60s and 70s.

As discussed above, the ASRM ethics committee discourages egg donation to women who are beyond the normal reproductive age because of concern for capacity of the "older" mother to medically, physically, and psychologically handle the possible multiple babies, as well as endure the social and parenting issues of raising a child.

Some of the emotional and ethical issues clinics grapple with include the following questions:

1. What is in the best interest for all involved—the donor, especially if she is a friend or family member, the intended parents, and potential offspring?

2. What underlies the motivations to pursue pregnancy?

3. Do we have the right to restrict access based on our own judgments?

4. Should we use available recipients for this population, rather than an eligible couple already on the waiting list?

5. Because of advanced age, should the clinic allow immediate access to the waiting list, thus restricting access to those already waiting?

Others argue that reproductive freedom is a constitutional right, even if it cannot occur "naturally" and the use of reproductive assistance is required. Historically, this argument is supported by case law; therefore, denying access to egg donation to postmenopausal women could be considered unconstitutional. In the adoption model, restriction is not necessarily based on age, but centers more around the welfare of the child and the provision for a healthy, supportive, and nurturing environment. Using the ethical standpoint of best interest of the child is a more non-discriminatory approach.

5. Why has sperm donation raised less complicated ethical issues than egg donation?

Sperm donation has been practiced for well over 200 years, and until HIV became a concern, the procedures for donor medical and genetic screening were very basic. Little attention was given to emotional and/or psychological considerations, social and family history, or to the long-term implications for the donor and/or recipient. In 1987, ASRM issued guidelines calling for a more standardized screening process for sperm donors in light of the concern of HIV and Hepatitis viruses and the potential for their transmission via donor insemination using fresh semen.

Also at this time, the application of IVF to include the use of donor eggs for infertile women was rapidly taking hold with the expansion of the donor pool to include anonymous donors. Because there are potential physical, medical, and psychological risks that donors will experience, a more uniform and rigorous physical, medical, and psychological screening protocol was developed as a necessary facet of a donor program.

In contrast to sperm donation, women who agree to donate their eggs are subjected to a medical intervention with the associated risks of ovarian hyperstimulation and anesthesia for egg retrieval performed under ultrasound guidance. Although a minor procedure, it is an invasive procedure and not without risk. Donor programs' guidelines recommend psychological testing, counseling, and informational sessions with a mental health professional as part of the screening process.

Published experience, as well as anecdotal experience of this author and colleagues, reveals a different finding in women who have conceived, delivered, and are parents through egg donation. Couples have reported less intense and ambivalent feelings when parenting through egg donation versus sperm donation. We believe this is because the mother established a biologic and emotional bond, as well as experienced pregnancy. Conversely, with the use of donor insemination, the husband has little or no necessary participation in a treatment cycle of donor insemination. This may only perpetuate the sense of estrangement that the father may feel from his potential offspring, if the issue is not addressed in the donor insemination counseling and screening appointment.

6. Who owns the embryos created in an IVF cycle and does that party have full authority as to their ultimate disposition?

In the absence of absolute law in most states, the individual for whom the embryos were created has ultimate decisional authority regarding the disposition of the embryos. However, this may be predicated on any institutional and clinic policy, and/or applicable state law. In the informed consent, before commencement of treatment, this policy or applicable law must be disclosed so that the individual's desires for disposition are in accordance with clinic policy and/or state law.

A complicated ethical issue may arise when embryos have been cryopreserved, the contract for continued storage expires, and repeated attempts to contact the "owners" of the embryos are unsuccessful. In this instance, after a predetermined period, the embryos may be considered "abandoned." Ownership may be transferred from the couple to the clinic, which may then have authority as to the ultimate disposition.

7. What are the options for those couples who elect not to use or continue storage of their cryopreserved embryos?

The embryos' ultimate destiny depends on individual state regulation and wishes of the couple, who have the primary right to make that decision. Informed consent issues arise from the potential uses of excess embryos. Should a couple elect not to use the frozen embryos, they must notify the clinic in writing requesting discontinuation of embryo storage. At that point, they again are asked to execute a legal statement as to their desired option for disposition. In most cases, couples that wish to discontinue storage of their embryos have achieved a pregnancy, delivered, and have completed their family.

Embryos may be disposed of in three ways unless otherwise directed by a written request. First, the embryos may be donated to another infertile couple after appropriate testing, screening, and counseling requirements are met. This may be a known or anonymous donation. Second, the embryos may be discarded in accordance with standard procedures and applicable legal requirements. Some couples may request that the embryos be thawed and be given to them so that they may dispose of them in a way comfortable for them. Finally, a couple may donate their embryos to the clinic, or another cryopreservation laboratory that might be conducting a specific embryo research protocol. Because the idea of embryo donation to another couple may be morally and/or ethically uncomfortable to them, the idea of donating their embryos to research makes them feel that they are contributing in gratitude.

8. What happens to frozen embryos if a marriage is dissolved due to either divorce or death of one or both partners?

As there is no law that governs the ultimate fate of cryopreserved embryos when any of these situations arise, the individual who elects to freeze any embryos must set forth in written instruction his/her desires for use and disposition of the embryos. Couples may have other directives or agreements aside from the three standard options described above. If so, outside legal counsel should be sought, and any directive should be attached to the clinic's executed legal statement. Finally, direction must be given for embryo disposition should the couple be unable to later agree on previously designated desires, or if they are unable to be contacted for storage contract renewal. The question that remains is whether the joint advance instructions for disposition of embryos will be legally binding when a divorce occurs, if one or both of the partners wish to deviate from the conditions previously set forth and the other does not concur.

9. Are there potential ethical issues for the patient and provider in treating women/couples with the ART, where one or both of the gamete donors have HIV?

Both the American College of Obstetrics and Gynecology (ACOG) (2003) and ASRM (2002) support, without reservation, the treatment of HIV discordant couples with reproductive assistance. It has been suggested by both that the risks involved in treating such couples do not exceed those of treating any other couple that may have a chronic disease or an unknown potential genetic predisposition that may be passed on to the offspring. In fact, there has been a suggestion that refusing HIV couples reproductive assistance, with the available data regarding safety, may in fact be a violation of the Americans With Disabilities Act (ADA).

Generally, an HIV-positive woman can use artificial insemination if she is otherwise fertile. An HIV-positive male may significantly reduce, but not completely eliminate, transmission to his female partner by using artificial insemination with rigorous sperm washing and processing techniques. The use of in vitro fertilization with intracytoplasmic sperm injection

(ICSI) has been suggested by some to further reduce the risk of HIV transmission. However, ongoing research in Europe and the United States has raised significant debate among providers as to whether it is necessary to use ICSI. The most recent research reveals artificial insemination with specialized sperm washing virtually eliminates the risk of horizontal transmission. In fact, some argue that exposing patients to the added physical, emotional, and financial drain of ART is unethical or a misuse of technology when there are other less aggressive therapies available.

10. *Case:* A couple with severe male factor infertility desire IVF treatment immediately following unsuccessful cycles of artificial insemination using her husband's sperm. They wanted to assess their fertilization potential prior to resorting to donor insemination. Twenty-four hours post-insemination of eight mature eggs, no fertilization was observed. The couple requests that the eggs now be inseminated with donor sperm so as not to "waste" the cycle. What is the ethical dilemma in this scenario?

In this situation, it is important to understand that the couple's frustration and grief over the result of no fertilization, coupled with their desperation that the cycle "not go to waste," supersedes the couple's ability to fully consider and be comfortable with the emotional sequelae that may accompany the use of donor sperm. ASRM Ethical Guidelines suggest that it is ethically acceptable to use donor sperm for IVF. However, it is strongly recommended that donor sperm should not be used during the initial IVF cycle attempt, when the woman's fertility is normal, but the man's fertilizing capacity is uncertain. Donor sperm should only be used when fertilization attempts with the husband's sperm have failed, and the execution of informed consent and appropriate counseling for donor sperm is done before the initiation of the IVF treatment.

In this instance, the ethical issue at the forefront is the knowledge of the treatment team that this couple has not resolved the male infertility issue and is not adequately prepared to consider the emotional and ethical ramifications of using donor sperm. Using donor sperm without adequate emotional and educational preparation would not be in the best interest of the couple, the potential offspring, and family.

11. What is the ethical concern in compensation for both sperm and egg donation programs?

Compensation is considered ethically acceptable for both egg and sperm donation. However, it should be based on the individual's time, risk assumed, and inconvenience incurred by coming for repeated office visits, screening, and diagnostic studies, as opposed to compensation being given for number or quality of eggs or sperm donated. Clearly, egg donors incur more time, risk, and inconvenience in the process of donating eggs than sperm donors. Therefore, there is more attention to the compensation issue in the egg donor arena.

ASRM addressed this issue out of concern for egg donation becoming too much like a commercial enterprise. The fear is that young women seeking participation may be more financially motivated, rather than altruistically. This could affect their commitment to the necessary treatment and compliance requirements. In the face of a very competitive climate, as programs expand their donor pools, there is additional concern that programs may minimize the recommended screening guidelines. They may also attempt to attract donors by offering higher than acceptable financial compensation. Finally, there are some couples offering additional compensation for personal and social characteristics, such as high I.Q. This is an ethical concern and is discouraged in a program's donor recruitment efforts.

12. *Case:* A couple who achieved success in the first IVF cycle where three embryos were replaced are diagnosed with a triplet pregnancy. It has been recommended that they undergo multi-fetal-reduction (MFR) to a twin pregnancy. The couple requests early chorionic villas testing (CVS) to determine the sex of the three fetuses in order to select the fetus to be terminated. Is it ethical to select gender in MFR?

Fetal reduction is a first-trimester procedure performed in the instance of a multiple gestation, usually triplet or greater, where the fetuses are assumed to be normal and the potential for medical harm is circumstantial. The intent of the reduction is to prevent the potential maternal and fetal complications secondary to multiple gestations and premature birth, not to terminate a pregnancy because of a known medical problem or anomaly such as in *selective termination*. In theory, then, fetal reduction can be ethically justified because it meets the ethical criteria of imposing the least harm with the most potential for good.

Doing a CVS, unless truly medically indicated, is also not recommended due to the challenge of trying to perform this procedure on a multiple gestation and the resulting increased potential for loss. In fetal reduction, there is not a "choice or selection" of the embryo to be reduced. General practice is to reduce the most accessible fetus or the one that has evidence of a potential abnormality.

The ethical position of most professional medical organizations is that no provider knowingly participates in gender selection for purely non-disease indications (personal, social, or cultural). This is not to suggest that some providers will never do the procedure for this purpose, but that a physician has the right to refuse to perform selective reduction for gender selection.

13. *Case:* **A couple wishes to conceive a child through IVF and pre-implantation selection of an embryo based on HLA compatibility with the recipient for the sole purpose of being an available donor for a sibling in need. Is it ethical to use this technology for this purpose?**

Pre-implantation genetic diagnosis (PGD) is a relatively new technology that offers the option of obtaining genetic information regarding an individual embryo prior to transfer to the uterus for potential implantation. If the embryos are to be created through IVF and exposed to PGD based on the sole intent of benefiting another—in this case, the sibling in need of an eligible bone marrow donor, there is ethical concern for the potential child being sought only as an instrument for the benefit of the sibling. It seems to be less ethically reprehensible when the parents present a dual motive for the desired pregnancy; they wish to find a suitable donor for their existing child, but have full intentions of pursuing the pregnancy regardless of whether they achieve an eligible HLA-matched embryo.

Aside from the ethical challenges presented by the procedure alone and the intent of the parents, there are additional ethical issues that should be addressed with the parents. They include the following:

1. Disposition of the non-matching embryos

2. Potential for only a few embryos available for PGD, lessening the likelihood of obtaining a match,

3. Potential for not achieving a successful pregnancy, and

4. Potential for the child in need dying before a successful pregnancy and birth is achieved.

14. *Case:* **A woman requests posthumous retrieval of sperm from her husband after his unexpected death in a motor vehicle accident. Why may this be ethically problematic?**

Historically, posthumous births have been recognized without legal or ethical question, as the conception would have occurred while the father was alive, and desire and consent is assumed. In this instance, the child is also assumed the legal child and heir of the deceased. Posthumous reproduction can be examined within the context of two different scenarios. First is a situation where an individual may actually contract to have sperm frozen prior to chemotherapy or radiation therapy to preserve his fertility potential. Second is a situation where there is an unexpected, sudden death and the wife or partner wishes to have sperm retrieved to achieve the pregnancy. The latter scenario presents the most ethical concerns for the reproductive specialist, as there is usually no consent of desire, intent, and/or consent of the deceased.

The author believes that a practitioner should not honor such a request to obtain sperm from a dying or deceased individual without evidence of informed consent, known desires, or specific direction from the donor for retrieval, storage, or use of his gametes after his death. Aside from whether such a practice is ethically acceptable, further ethical challenges regarding survivor benefits of the potential offspring must also be taken into consideration.

15. *Case:* A couple is concerned that their potential off-spring conceived with donor insemination may later marry another conceived with the same donor. What ethical issues arise concerning the potential for consanguinity in the use of donor sperm or donor eggs?

Prior to 1987 when donor insemination was performed with fresh semen, most practices providing this service screened their own donors and processed fresh donor semen obtained on the day of the artificial insemination. Now it is mandatory for all donor sperm to be screened for HIV and other infectious disease, quarantined for 6 months and released for use only after donor rescreening is obtained. Therefore, most practices refer couples to well-established sperm banks for donor selection.

ASRM Guidelines for Gamete and Embryo Donation (2002) suggested that limiting the number of pregnancies resulting from an individual sperm donor to 10 would virtually eliminate the potential for consanguinity from a particular donor. As there is no imposed regulation concerning the number of pregnancies with an individual donor, it is incumbent on the sperm bank to observe the ASRM ethical guideline limiting the number to 10 pregnancies.

Conforming to these ASRM Guidelines requires accurate recording and follow-up of all pregnancies established. This may be well controlled in an onsite cryopreservation program, but is more difficult when multiple facilities are employed. Sperm banks service the nation and worldwide so it is thought unlikely that consanguinity would be as much of an issue as it may have been in the past where the individual donor's sperm was being used in a comparatively small geographic area.

16. **What is the difference between a "traditional surrogate" and an IVF gestational carrier?**

The concept of gestational carrier is a natural extension of the IVF process allowing couples the option of having their own biologic child. It is appropriate for infertile women, who are genetically sound, but unable to carry a pregnancy due to

1. congenital absence or surgical removal of the uterus;

2. a reproductively impaired uterus, myomas, uterine synechiae, or any other congenital abnormalities; or

3. a medical condition, that might be life-threatening during pregnancy, such as diabetes, immunologic problems, or severe heart, kidney, or liver disease.

In the gestational carrier procedure, the genetic mother undergoes the ovulation induction and egg retrieval phases of IVF. The eggs are inseminated with her husband's sperm, and once normal embryo development has occurred, the embryos are placed in a woman who has contracted to carry the child. This must be distinguished from surrogate motherhood, wherein the surrogate mother is inseminated with the sperm of the husband of the infertile woman and, thus, has a genetic contribution to the child. In the carrier relationship, the carrier has no genetic investment in the child.

Ethical issues for both traditional surrogacy and IVF gestational surrogacy are similar in many ways. Some of the questions to consider include

1. What will happen if the baby is malformed or unwanted by the surrogate mother or the contracting couple?

2. What happens if there is a death of either or both of the commissioning parents or they separate or divorce during the surrogate pregnancy?

3. Is it ethical to allow a woman who may have a disabling medical disease or congenital reproductive problem to pass this trait to her potential offspring?

4. As the commercialization of surrogacy becomes commonplace, how will we stop the exploitation of poor and minority women by for-profit agencies recruiting candidates for couples?

5. What is the impact on surrogate or carrier's children as they experience a child being born of their mother, and then given away?

For both surrogacy and gestational carrier options the ASRM Guidelines recommend that it is unethical to consider using surrogacy or gestational carrier for purely social or non-medical reasons, such as convenience for a woman who does not wish to undergo pregnancy.

There has been more ethical concern given to the practice of surrogate motherhood due to negative public opinion and misunderstanding generated about the surrogacy, with the famous Marybeth Whitehead case (Baby M) that occurred in New Jersey in the late 1980s. The contract between Marybeth Whitehead, the surrogate, and the Stearns, the infertile couple, was deemed invalid because it violated New Jersey state law regarding adoption. Although there continues to be an absence of law regarding such contracts, it is assumed that they are not binding. These contracts serve as a means of good faith and intent between the commissioning couple and the surrogate or carrier couple.

The ASRM distinguished between the ethical concerns of these two options and recommendations for their use. The ASRM had more reservations regarding the use of surrogacy and recommended a limited use of surrogacy because of the legal risks, ethical concerns, and potential physical and psychological effects. Gestational carriers appear to be more willing to be IVF mothers because of the elimination of genetic component and opportunity to undertake a purely altruistic endeavor.

17. Who is considered the "mother" in circumstances where couples have used such applied IVF technologies as donor oocytes and gestational surrogacy?

When a third party enters into the reproductive process either as a gamete or embryo donor, or a gestational carrier, the concept of "collaborative" mother becomes increasingly complex. It is possible to have an egg and/or sperm donor, embryo donor, and/or a gestational carrier/surrogate and finally, the rearing parents. Creating a new definition of mother, father, or parent has lagged far behind the reality of these alternatives.

In the case of the woman who uses an egg donor, there is no genetic investment, but the recipient is the gestational and rearing parent. If the egg donor is anonymous, or known, the question is who is considered "the mother"? Although only five states have specific law defining the egg donor recipient as the legal mother, other states have adopted the uniform stance, which is, the mother is the one who delivers the child.

If we assume the legal mother is the woman who gives birth to the child, some legal and ethical considerations exist in the case of IVF gestational surrogacy and traditional surrogacy arrangements. In the arena of gestational IVF surrogacy, the biologic or genetic parents have had to petition the courts to name the genetic parents as the parents to be listed on the birth certificate, despite the gestational carrier being the one to deliver the child.

Conversely, in traditional surrogacy in which the woman who delivers the child is also the genetic mother, the distinction is less clear. In the majority of states, the surrogate is considered the mother for legal and all other purposes. After the birth, she can decide to follow through with the pre-conceptual contract with the commissioning parents and continue the process for relinquishing the child.

18. Should women newly diagnosed with cancer be offered the option to preserve their fertility pre-chemo or radiation therapy by cryopreservation of oocytes (research protocol) or isolation of ovarian tissue for cryopreservation?

There is strong consensus among cancer survivors that it is an ethical obligation for medical and surgical oncologists to inform men and women of the detrimental effect of chemo and radiation therapy on potential fertility. Cancer itself, as well as chemo and radiation therapy, can affect fertility through its major cellular and physiological impact on gonadal function causing germ cell depletion.

Pre-treatment options for women who want to preserve fertility include the following:

1. Immediate IVF and cryopreservation of resulting embryos for later potential use.

2. Experimental oocyte cryopreservation, where mature eggs are retrieved after induction of ovulation and frozen for later use. At present, it offers only a 3% pregnancy rate at best.

3. Experimental ovarian tissue freezing involves removal of the ovary by laparoscopy and cryopreservation for later transplantation in the woman's body. At present, there has been approximately 50% restoration of ovarian and hormonal function, at least temporarily, with no pregnancies to date.

One ethical challenge is preserving fertility for this population and not causing harm by delaying necessary chemo or radiation therapy. For instance, it may not be in the best interest for a woman with a steroid dependent cancer to undergo IVF, because of the elevated estrogen levels that result from ovarian stimulation.

Another ethical concern is offering these latter two unproven and experimental procedures to the oncology community or potential subjects. Full disclosure of the experimental nature of these procedures, their potential for success, current limitations, and hope for future use should be fully disclosed. Current recommendations of ASRM are that these procedures be under the continued review and approval of an Institutional Review Board. Finally, if the oocytes were not used, the disposal of them carries less ethical concern than that of stored embryos.

19. What resources are available for professionals working with patients who are undergoing fertility treatment?

Educational support and continuing education opportunities are available through ASRM and ACOG, both of which have special interest groups on assisted reproduction. Several pharmaceutical companies also have a strong commitment to both professional and patient information and education. For instance, Serono, Organon, and Ferring, manufacturers of fertility drugs, all host annual nursing conferences, addressing provision of care in the reproductive endocrinology and infertility field. In a field where information is "old news" by the time it is published, the ability to have collegial and anecdotal information and support at one's disposal through networking with nursing colleagues is invaluable.

To help professionals deal with the ever-changing technologies and confront the never ending ethical challenges that arise, most programs or clinics form a multidisciplinary ethics committee. Included on such a committee are legal counsel, mental health professionals, physicians, nurses, and embryologists. If possible, an obstetrical consultant and geneticist and/or genetics nurse counselor are also included. These committees are composed of interested members of the IVF team who are responsible for reviewing issues or cases that arise and then bringing relevant information and recommendations to the team at large for discussion or resolution. Advising a couple that a particular request cannot be honored because of ethical concerns is much easier when the case has been brought to the ethics committee for review and discussion. Many university-based programs have a hospital ethics committee that may be involved.

RESOURCES

American College of Obstetrics and Gynecology. (2003). *Ethics in obstetrics and gynecology: Human immunodeficiency virus: Ethical guidelines for obstetricians and gynecologists.* Washington, DC: Author.

American Society for Reproductive Medicine. (2002). The minimum guidelines for in vitro fertilization and gamete donation programs and ethical considerations of the assisted reproductive technologies. In *2002 guidelines for gamete and embryo donation*. Retrieved from http://www.asrm.org

Center for Bioethics at the University of Pennsylvania. www.bioethics.upenn.edu

Ethics Committee of the American Society of Reproductive Medicine. (2002). Human immunodeficiency virus and infertility treatment. *Fertility and Sterility*, 7(2), 218–222.

Practice Committee of the American Society for Reproductive Medicine & Society for Assisted Reproductive Technology. (2003). Revised minimum standards for practice offering assisted reproductive technologies. *Fertility and Sterility*, 80(6), 1556–1559.

Chapter 8

Ethical Issues in the Care of Neonates and Infants

Anne M. Lovell

1. What is the nurse's obligation or recourse when he/she believes that the neonatologist is not providing adequate information to parents?

The neonatal intensive care unit (NICU) nurse may recognize these questions as "everyday" ethical issues, given the number and variety of caregivers involved with seriously ill neonates. It is the ethical duty of all healthcare professionals caring for a patient to communicate with the parents or guardians so that they can truly be informed and fully consent to all treatment. The NICU nurse is in a unique position to facilitate conversation between and among physicians, and to inform them quite directly what parents do not know or understand. The nurse is frequently the person to whom the parents look for help in understanding complicated medical information. In the case of genuine withholding of information, or information conflict, the nurse should assist in empowering the parents toward more open communication, protecting their autonomy as decision makers for the infant. Assistance could also be provided by patient representatives in this regard.

2. What is the nurse's obligation when the physician is not being truthful with parents about the infant's prognosis?

Ethically, the nurse's role is to support the parents, and help provide an environment in which they may feel safe and confident in the care that is being provided to their infant. If the nurse believes that the physician is withholding information or shading the truth regarding treatment or prognosis, the nurse first needs to speak to the physician, in order to fully understand the information upon which the physician is basing statements to the parents. Sometimes both clinicians and parents have a psychological interest in maintaining a mutual charade that medicine is all powerful. Some clinicians are reluctant to reveal the uncertainties of medicine to parents, fearing that it may undermine the parent's faith in the physician's knowledge and ability. However, research repeatedly shows that most people want the truth, no matter how painful it may be to hear.

In a situation in which discussing the issue with the physician does not resolve the concern, the nurse would want to investigate ways in which the parents could be correctly informed without damaging trust in their infant's caregivers. This would likely include speaking to a nursing supervisor and perhaps asking for an ethics consultation.

3. When care appears futile, is the nurse obligated to carry out orders that are painful or harmful to the infant?

According to the ANA *Code of Ethics for Nurses*, "Nurses may express their conscientious objections to participation . . . whenever possible, such a refusal should be made in advance and in time for alternative arrangements to be made for patient care . . . to avoid patient abandonment, and to withdraw only when assured that alternative sources of nursing care are available to the patient" (*Code for Nurses*).

A nurse should not be obligated to provide care in conflict with the nurse's value system, and probably would choose to work in an institution or patient care area where this is unlikely to occur. If such a situation does occur, if the nurse is the most experienced to provide care in a specific instance, or if staffing does not permit re-assignment, the nurse must provide the best and most compassionate care at the time it is required. Then, as soon as feasible, the nurse must address the issue. Two possible outcomes of action in bringing the issue to the attention of supervisors are reconsideration of the infant's treatment (in light of ultimate benefit versus present burden) or that the nurse would not be required to continue to provide care for that particular infant.

4. How much weight should be given to parents' wishes or demands regarding the type of care given to their baby?

Parents have traditionally been considered appropriate surrogate decision makers for their children. In the absence of evidence to the contrary, healthcare professionals usually do not question parents' rights to make healthcare decisions. However, this right is not absolute. If a conflict occurs between medical caregivers and parents, it can usually be resolved by education of the parents regarding the reasons for the recommendations, and of the caregivers regarding the parents' viewpoint. In the instance when standard of care medical treatment for a child is refused by parents, an ethics consultation is in order. If this is unsuccessful in achieving resolution, then legal advice and action may be sought by physicians and institutions.

5. How should a nurse handle situations that involve unusual or bizarre requests or activities that are consistent with parents' spiritual or cultural beliefs, but may be harmful or counterproductive to the infant's care?

To deal successfully with another's culture, the nurse must first appreciate his/her own emotions and biases. When a family makes an unusual request, the nurse should first evaluate whether the action or practice is consistent with good care for the infant. If it is not, perhaps a compromise can be reached to allow the family to do something else, which would be safe for the infant. If the action is safe and reasonable, but there is concern about offending staff or other families, the way to address this is to engage a nurse, physician, social worker, or pastoral care associate who would be able to support the family, and then to arrange for privacy for their activities. If this is not possible, justice would demand that an unusual request from one family not disrupt care in the NICU in general, or engender anxiety in other parents.

6. Is it ethical to expect/require families with limited financial, emotional, and/or intellectual resources to continue to deliver high-tech care of a compromised infant in the home?

NICU nurses may feel conflicted when a fragile newborn is discharged home with complicated care needs that previously were provided exclusively in an intensive care setting. Involvement in discharge planning provides an opportunity for the nurse to raise questions and concerns if the nurse thinks that the family is unwilling or unable to provide appropriate care. Even with optimal support, home care may not be safe for the infant or may stretch the limits of the family to a breaking point. The primary nurse, working in collaboration with a case manager, is in a position to raise and help resolve these practical and ethical concerns.

7. What does the primary nurse say when the family asks, "What do you think about this recommendation? What would you do if this were your baby"?

This query may be reframed as not *whether* to answer the question, but *how*. In this type of situation, there is a tension for the nurse between "what would I want to know if it were my child, what do I think *they* want to know, and what do *I want them to know*." So the dilemma seems to be "what is this parent really asking me?" Most importantly, it is vital to recognize that the question demands an answer, one which is more insightful than, "this is not my child, so I cannot tell you what to do." It is essential that advice-seeking parents not perceive abandonment by healthcare providers.

Some parents may want to be told what to do, but more likely, they are really requesting a conversation. The nurse could ask, "What frightens you most about making this decision?" This type of interaction can provide the opportunity for the nurse to discuss values, and the context in which a decision is to be made, considering the possible outcomes for all concerned. Ideally, the nurse assists the parents in their role as autonomous decision makers for the baby, without placing him/herself into their situation.

8. Is it permissible to "bend the rules" for more liberal visitation in the NICU?

First of all, what are the rules of the NICU? If they are very strict (for instance, only allowing parents to visit with restrictive time limits), it would be appropriate to investigate when and why the policies were made, and what the appropriate channels are to initiate a review and revision. Most children's hospitals and special care nurseries pride themselves on a family-centered care model, with liberal visiting for babies and children.

If, however, the NICU already has liberal or "open" visiting for parents, and other family members are allowed, then any other requests would be dependent upon several factors. Decisions should be based upon hospital policy, the condition of the infant, the agreement of the family (they may not all agree with the request), and any additional burden to the staff or other families in allowing the NICU visitation.

9. *Case:* The parents have requested that a school-age child be allowed to bathe, dress, and hold her recently deceased infant sibling. Most of the staff are

very uncomfortable with this request—what is the best response to my colleagues?

There appear to be two questions or concerns here: the nurses may be uncomfortable with this unusual request, from both the perspective of their own discomfort, and they may also be worried about the effect on the sibling. A response should be based upon several factors: the chronological and developmental age of the child and his/her relationship with the infant and the anticipated response of the child and family during the time the baby's body is being prepared in this way. On the one hand, this type of grieving and acceptance of death may be consistent with the family's values and/or culture, and represent a positive first step for them in dealing with the death; alternatively, if it is the parents' idea, and the child is reluctant or frightened, it should be discouraged. If done, a private place should be provided, away from other families.

10. *Case:* **A baby with a "lethal" genetic condition is transferred to the NICU. His parents had expected a stillborn infant, or a baby who would die in the delivery room. The family is now faced with treatment decisions they did not expect. How should the nurse support the family and answer their questions about what they may perceive as inaccurate information or guidance?**

Parents may be counseled, either prenatally, or shortly after birth, that their infant has a lethal condition. For example, babies who have Trisomy 13 or Trisomy 18 are often said to have lethal conditions, and most die in the neonatal period from associated anomalies. However, some children with these chromosome abnormalities live for 6–12 months, and occasionally longer. Parents may be approached regarding surgical procedures, or assisted ventilation. It is very important to ensure that parents receive consistent and accurate information regarding exactly what a physician means by "lethal," what that means for their child in particular, and if there are any treatment options to consider. If there are conflicts between caregivers and parents, in terms of requesting or refusing treatment, an ethics consultation may be indicated.

11. What are the ethical issues surrounding a staff nurse who becomes attached to an infant in the NICU, and then is able to circumvent normal or usual processes to adopt that baby?

It is not unusual for nurses to have special feelings for certain babies in the NICU. However, professionalism dictates that the nurse must always recognize that there are boundaries in the nurse/patient relationship, even if they are not always well-defined. The ANA (2001) *Code of Ethics* states, "The intimate nature of nursing care . . . present(s) the potential for blurring of limits to professional relationships. Maintaining authenticity and expressing oneself as an individual, while remaining within the bounds established by the purpose of the relationship, can be especially difficult in prolonged or long-term relationships. When those professional boundaries are jeopardized the nurse should seek assistance from peers or supervisors or take the appropriate steps to remove her/himself from the situation" (American Nurses Association, 2001, p. 11). The nurse's adoptive home might be the best placement for the baby, but this cannot be appropriately evaluated if normal procedures for adoption are not observed. Beneficence and justice dictates that all available placements should be evaluated prior to placing the baby.

12. *Case:* One of the NICU nurses has become "territorial" about an infant; she buys clothes for her, and questions the parents' visitation practices, their attachment to the infant, and their actual/potential ability to care for her. Also, she criticizes other staff caring for the infant in her absence. What is the role or obligation of the nurse's colleagues/coworkers?

The primary concern in this instance would seem to be the issue of dual relationship, where the nurse has crossed professional boundaries and is considering the infant emotionally "her baby" while still functioning as the nurse. NICU nurses appreciate that parent-infant bonding may be impaired when an infant is very ill and often technology dependent. A vital role of the nurse is to facilitate bonding and familiarity, and educate the parents in the baby's care, rather than threaten or alienate them by her attitude or actions. A professional medical relationship (in this case, between nurse and parent) is one of unequal power. It is ethically wrong for the nurse to take advantage of her "power" of knowing more about the infant's condition and care and having greater access to the baby. The primary nurse should be reminded of her role by colleagues, and possibly counseled by a supervisor. The best solution may be to reassign this infant to another primary nurse.

13. Is it ethically acceptable for a nurse to accept personal gifts from parents of an infant whom she has cared for over a period of weeks or months, or to socialize with them outside the NICU, either prior to the baby's discharge, or after (e.g., at a birthday or christening party for the child)?

Families often wish to show appreciation to nurses who have had a special role in their child's care, but this again reflects a difficult professional boundary issue. A gift by definition does not imply reciprocation, but it is impossible to truly know the motive for gift giving in a professional relationship. If families insist, they should be encouraged to show their appreciation with an impersonal gift that can be shared—for instance, bringing a homemade treat for the entire unit, or giving a donation for books for the NICU waiting area.

Dual relationships (professional and personal) with families may cause problems related to treatment decisions or issues of care if a nurse is emotionally close to a family. Other families who observe a "special relationship" between a nurse and family may feel resentful or wonder if another baby is receiving better care than their own infant.

14. What are the "Baby Doe" rules?

The "Baby Doe" Regulations are the final result of a situation in 1982 when a baby with Trisomy 21 (Down syndrome) was born with a surgically repairable birth defect. His parents elected to withhold surgical treatment, and allow the baby to die, based upon his prognosis of mental retardation, citing the financial and emotional burden on the family. This child came to be known as Baby Doe, and his death started a cascade of legal actions and ethical debates regarding provision of treatment to neonates with very serious physical and/or mental impairments. The final Baby Doe Regulations state that life-sustaining treatment must be provided to all disabled newborns with the following exceptions:

a. The infant is chronically and irreversibly comatose;

b. Provision of such treatment would merely prolong dying or not be effective in ameliorating or correcting the infant's life-threatening conditions;

c. Provision of such treatment would be virtually *futile* (in terms of survival) and the treatment itself under such circumstances would be *inhumane*.

15. How can nurses help parents struggling with decisions surrounding their critically ill infants?

It is possible for parents to decline treatment for their infant without conflicting with the "Baby Doe" model. Many ethicists believe that it is appropriate to consider quality of life issues when making treatment decisions.

If an infant's prognosis is favorable, the ethical principle of beneficence guides the professional to assist the parents to make treatment decisions, and to help them care for and bond with the infant. If the prognosis is grim or virtually hopeless, in terms of meaningful survival, non-maleficence dictates that comfort care of the infant, and support during parental grieving is most important. In the "gray" area, when an infant is very ill or impaired, and prognosis is uncertain, parents must be educated, and encouraged to become decision makers in collaboration with the healthcare providers. Truth-telling and autonomy are the guiding ethical principles here, as the caregivers guide the parents through complicated medical information, keep them clearly informed of potential success of treatments and realistic burdens, and optimally allow them to be decision makers at this difficult time.

16. What should a nurse do when parents have made a decision that the nurse thinks is ethically wrong?

First, consider the role of the primary nurse in this situation. If the parents, the physician(s), and possibly a spiritual advisor have come to this difficult decision, and they are as comfortable as possible with their choice, then there may be no ethical dilemma at all. "Ethical distress" is a situation in which someone is prevented from implementing or suggesting a decision one "feels" or "knows" is right. The individual may wish to intervene in the decision making, but has no personal authority and/or no access to decision-making channels. The nurse may truly believe that a wrong decision has been made, but it is not the nurse's decision. The nurse's beliefs and feelings should not be discounted, but should not be imposed upon the parents. It may be advisable for the nurse to request a change of assignment, and allow another nurse to care for the baby. The nurse may also wish to speak to a member of the hospital Ethics Committee, but should think carefully before requesting a formal consult, if she is the only person in conflict with the decision.

17. What should a nurse say when an extremely premature infant is transferred to the NICU from the delivery room *against the parents wishes and prior directive*?

This is obviously not a nursing decision, but the nurse can assist the father (and eventually the mother) to understand that not all resuscitation decisions can be made prenatally. The parents may feel betrayed and angry if they believed a plan had been agreed upon before the birth, and is now not being honored. However, if birth weight is higher than anticipated, or the infant appears more mature and vigorous than predicted by gestational date, the physicians may be compelled to treat that infant until more information is learned about the infant's condition. It is important that the parents be told that treatment decisions may be made every day, dependent upon the progress or decline of the infant's condition. The nurse may help facilitate this type of education and conversation between parent and physician, in the hope that they will be able to work together in assessing benefits and burdens of continuing treatment for the infant.

18. *Case:* **I have been taking care of a baby for 3 months in the NICU. He is almost ready to be discharged to home, although his prognosis is very grim for long-term survival, due to congenital and acquired problems. His parents are requesting a minor "cosmetic" procedure prior to discharge. The surgeon is willing to do this, but I think it is unethical to put the baby through another surgery. What can I do?**

This is another question where the ethical answer is largely dependent upon the benefits and burdens of the specific treatment for the infant. First, you may want to speak with the surgeon in order to understand what the surgery entails, and why the parents are requesting it. Is the procedure entirely cosmetic or might there be a modicum of benefit for the baby? As an example, a surgical procedure to correct an eye muscle problem may not be necessary for vision in a child who is predicted to die within a few months. However, the burden (in terms of anesthesia risk, surgical risk, and post-operative pain) may be relatively low, while the emotional benefit to the parents in relating to and nurturing their child may be a significant benefit for both. If the benefit appears to clearly outweigh the burden (risk and pain), then it would seem that this was a carefully considered decision by parents and providers. In that case, continuing care of the infant and support of the parents are in order.

19. What if the parents don't agree on major decisions?

Unless one parent clearly and legally has been awarded the decision-making authority for the infant, both parents' feelings and decisions must be considered. In these types of situations, members of the Ethics Committee of the institution may be asked to consult, and their primary role is often to provide a forum for discussion of competing interests regarding care decisions. If, despite continuing education and discussion about the infant's condition, the parents still cannot arrive at a mutual decision, the care team may agree to maintain life support until the infant's condition changes, or the parents are able to agree. This is a situation when it is often valuable to seek the advice and support of the institution's Risk Management Department.

20. *Case:* **The healthcare team has recommended a very complicated heart surgery for a baby in the NICU, and the family will almost certainly agree, in an effort to save their baby. I know, from previous experience, that another institution has done many more of these procedures, and has a higher success rate in infants. Should I tell the family?**

This family has been presented with an extremely difficult situation, and the ethical principle of non-maleficence would caution that no additional psychological burden be added. However, beneficence would seem to demand that every effort be made to give the baby the best chance of survival. The autonomy of the parents may also be at risk for compromise if they are not given all options for making this life or death decision for their child. Several issues must be considered:

1. Is it truly feasible for the family to consider another institution, relative to their resources and the ability to travel and stay in another location? Would transfer to another facility present hardships such as a parent losing a job, or child care for siblings? Could these be managed?

2. Is it in the best interest of the infant to be transported to another facility? Is the surgery emergent or elective? How much time can be "bought" for this infant before the surgery?

3. Are all the facts of the case known to the nurse? Perhaps transfer has already been considered and rejected for medical or psychosocial reasons.

If the above issues have been addressed, and the nurse still believes that not all options have been presented to the family, the nurse would be wise to discuss these concerns with the managing physician and/or supervisor, prior to sharing these concerns with the family.

RESOURCES

American Nurses Association. (2001). *Code of ethics for nurses with interpretive statements, provision 2.4*. Washington, DC: American Nurses Publishing.

Boyle, R. J. (1997). Decisions about treatment for newborns, infants and children. In J. Fletcher, P. Lombardo, M. Marshall, & F. Miller (Eds.), *Introduction to clinical ethics* (2nd ed., pp. 181–204). Hagerstown, MD: University Publishing Group, Inc.

Emedicine. Clinical knowledge base in neonatology. www.emedicine.com/ped/NEONATOLOGY.htm

Frankel, C. A., & Juengst, E. T. (1991). Cosmetic surgery for a fatally ill infant. *Journal of Pediatric Ophthalmology and Strabismus, 28*(5), 250–254.

Hulac, P. (2001). Creation and use of *You Are Not Alone*, a video for parents facing difficult decisions. *The Journal of Clinical Ethics, 12*(3), 251–253.

Koogler, T., Wilfond, B., & Ross, L. F. (2003). Lethal language, lethal decisions. *Hastings Center Report, 33*(2), 37–41.

National Association of Neonatal Nurses. www.nann.org

Neonatal Network. www.neonatalnetwork.com

Paris, J. J., Ferranti, J., & Reardon, F. (2001). From the Johns Hopkins Baby to Baby Miller: What have we learned from four decades of reflection on neonatal cases? *The Journal of Clinical Ethics, 12*(3), 207–214.

Purtillo, R. (1980). Competing ethical values in medicine. *New England Journal of Medicine, 303*(25), 1482.

Ross, L. F. (2003). Why, 'Doctor, if this were your child, what would you do?' deserves an answer. *The Journal of Clinical Ethics, 14*(1/2), 59–62.

Ruddick, W. (2003). Answering parents' questions. *The Journal of Clinical Ethics, 14*(1/2), 68–78.

Chapter 9

Ethical Issues in the Care of Children

Lauren G. McAliley

1. How can I prepare children for receiving shots?

How should the nurse respond to the following?

- The parent tells the child that the shot won't hurt.

- The parent laughs when the child cries and says, "Wait until I tell Billy you cried like a baby."

- The parent says, "Now she's gonna give you a shot—that's what you get for being so bad."

Honesty, sensitivity, and promotion of the child's comfort and self-esteem are primary considerations. These objectives can often be accomplished by modeling alternative responses that don't appear to directly contradict the parent. In situations where that doesn't seem possible, contradicting the parent is less morally objectionable than misleading the child, generating mistrust of healthcare professionals or damaging his/her ego. Try the following:

- "Some people tell me it pinches, some tell me it hurts a little, some say it tickles, and some even say they hardly felt anything at all. You can tell me what it feels like to you when we are all done."

- "Did you know that lots of kids and even some grownups say ouch or cry when they get shots? You did a good job because you stopped crying pretty quickly and you tried to hold still even though it hurt. THAT takes courage!"

- "Your Mom is just teasing, isn't she? She knows that we don't give shots to people because they were bad. She knows we give shots to people so they don't get sick and have to stay in the hospital."

2. **Case: A 6-year-old child with leukemia and neutropenia is misbehaving to the point of being disruptive to other patients and the staff. Her parents won't discipline her because "she's been through so much." How can we intervene?**

   Some acting out is to be expected and may be an important part of coping, but children with serious illness still need structure and limits. Behavior that is disruptive to the child's treatment or to others is clearly unacceptable. The following may be helpful.

   - Child Life Specialist, Social Worker or Psychologist assessment of child and family—are there special psychological factors/needs?

   - Provide child with age appropriate diversions and give choices/permit control over treatment and routine as much as possible.

   - Meet with family to explain need for behavioral limits; identify those behaviors that can be ignored and those that are unacceptable; discuss appropriate responses to misbehavior; emphasize need for praise and reward when behaving well. Natural consequences, time-outs, sticker charts (a calendar representing days or hours on which stickers are placed when a child successfully avoided or accomplished a predetermined behavior), loss of toys/privileges, earning of extra toys/privileges may all be useful.

   - Meet with child to discuss expectations, consequences, and rewards and, as possible, involve her in making some of the decisions.

   - Ensure all staff and family are aware of and consistently enforce the above (an explicit care plan would be helpful).

- Sometimes formal contracting with parents/child may be necessary.

3. *Case:* **There is a 14-year-old who will likely die of cystic fibrosis (CF) within days or weeks or, at most, months. He has been here when other patients with CF died and was once in the intensive care unit on a ventilator for a brief period. He wants a do not resuscitate (DNR) order in case he arrests but the parents are insisting on full resuscitation efforts. Is it ethical to support the patient's choice even though he is a minor?**

    By default, parents make medical decisions on behalf of their minor children, but this parental right and duty is not without limits. As children mature, an increasing amount of weight must be given to their preferences. The hospital legal department may have something to say about the actions ultimately taken by the healthcare team, but the ethics of the situation support advocating for and acting in keeping with this minor patient's wishes.

    - By age 14, most children understand the permanence, universality, and inevitability of death (this should be confirmed in this patient's case).

    - This child has had experiences with the deaths of other patients with CF and likely understands the causality of death (should be confirmed).

    - This child has lived with the burdens of CF and experienced life in the intensive care unit hooked up to a ventilator—he can appreciate these experiences in a way his parents cannot.

    - Death is inevitable in the near future and resuscitation will, if successful, prolong the process of dying. It may, in fact, be perceived by the child as dying more than once.

An ethics committee meeting with parents present and/or some counseling may be helpful in convincing the parents to support their child's choice. The parents may need concrete advice about how to have (and handle emotionally) such sensitive discussions with the child.

4. *Case:* **The parents of an anencephalic 4-year-old child have made the agonizing decision to stop nutrition and fluids, knowing death could take several days to occur. The nurses caring for the dying child feel the need to play music, rock her, and talk to her just as they would any other patient. Because this confused the parents and made them question their decision, the attending physician wants the nurses to stop. What do we do when the coping practices of the nurses cause conflict for the family?**

The physician writes the orders but does not establish an ongoing presence with the child. The nurses (along with the family) will provide the care until death ensues. Most pediatric nurses outside of the intensive care units and the oncology setting do not have experience working with the imminently dying child. Despite what science tells us about what an anencephalic child does or does not experience, it seems counterintuitive from an emotional perspective to withhold the human touches we traditionally offer out of respect for the dignity of the individual (and often, out of concern for the family's sensitivities as well). Providing this attention to the child allows the nurses to "care" and to cope.

The nurses must be given some insight as to how their coping measures influence the family and an attempt should be made to help the family understand the nurses' position. The family may identify with the needs of the staff and, thus, find their ministrations acceptable. If the family remains confused or upset, the nurses should stop as requested by the physician. In that case, it should be made clear what care is acceptable and opportunities should be put in place for staff to share the care responsibilities, debrief their experience, and grieve the death of the patient.

5. What is my responsibility when I hear or see a parent disciplining a patient or a patient's sibling with a belt?

Parents have the right and responsibility to instill values and to discipline their children so those children become civilized and functional members of society. However, children are not property and there are limits to parental authority.

Extreme/Damaging   Permissiveness
Physical Unbounded
or Emotional Discipline

ABUSE   **NEGLECT**

"Spanking" (on the buttocks with the flat of the hand), if used judiciously, won't seriously hurt the child. However, it may convey the sense that problems can be solved with violence and may confuse the child who is being taught that it is wrong to hit.

"Beating" a child (hitting with closed fist, striking with an object, hitting parts of the body other than the seat of the pants, or spanking with such force that bruises or permanent marks are caused) is thought by most professionals to be unacceptable. Between two adults, beating would constitute legally punishable activity. "Beating" is thought to be excessive and there is a risk of serious unintended injury if the child moves or the parent loses control.

Nurses have an obligation to intervene when a child is being beaten but to do so is uncomfortable and not entirely without risk.

- One approach is to focus on the needs of the parent. "You've been here all day and I can see little Bobby is quite a handful. Would you like me to get something for him to do and something for you to drink?" Then, when mother and child are calm, indicate that you would like to talk about some forms of discipline that can be very helpful. Offer pamphlets and an opportunity to talk with a Child Life Specialist or Social Worker.

- If the parent is confrontational, "Mind your own business. I'm his mother and I'll discipline him any way I choose," be matter-of-fact in stating that you are obligated by policy and law to report discipline that seems out of control or abusive and you don't want to have to do that. Tell her you can see she is frustrated and you believe she is well intended but she has to find another way to discipline her child than to beat him with a belt. Offer same choices as above.

- Assess for other behaviors (or physical findings) that suggest a hospital social worker consult or a mandated report to public children's services agency or police is in order.

6. *Case:* **A 3-year-old patient is ready for discharge. Her mother just arrived to pick her up. She is acting normally but there is a strong smell of alcohol about her. What should I do?**

We are obligated to make reasonably sure we are discharging children to environments where their general and medical needs can be safely met. In this case, there is the immediate concern about the ability to drive safely and the broader concern about possible alcoholism and risk for child neglect or abuse. An assessment needs to be made by a nurse, physician, or social worker.

- Is it truly alcohol that the nurse smells? Get a second person's opinion and if that person agrees, confront directly, "I detect a strong smell of alcohol and I am concerned about you driving right now." The parent's response must be carefully evaluated along with any evidence that the parent is impaired in any way.
- Is this parent driving or is someone else actually driving, and, if so, is that person sober?
- If there appears to be a legitimate safety concern, would the parent accept a cab voucher, arrange for someone else to come get them, or agree to wait a few hours before driving home?
- Evidence of impairment, belligerence/defensiveness, or a dubious story may warrant delay in discharge and require involvement of the physician, and possibly a social worker and/or Security. A report to a public children's service agency may be warranted as well— particularly if there are other indicators of neglect such as failure-to-thrive, inappropriate parent/child interactions, failure to keep medical appointments, or obtain immunizations.

7. **What do I do when a patient or family asks for an update about another child and I know that the two families have always shared detailed information openly?**

"Respect for persons" or the "autonomy" principle inspires the obligation to preserve privacy and confidentiality. Patients and families may choose to disclose whatever they wish but their disclosure practices don't constitute consent for us to disclose similarly. In this scenario you might try the following: "Federal law and hospital policy don't permit us to share information about other patients and families. It's perfectly natural for you to care and I'm sure (the patient) would appreciate your concern but I hope you'll understand that I can't answer." It is important not to make the questioner feel he/she has violated any standard. It sometimes backfires to add, "we take your own privacy just as seriously" because many families will add, "oh, we don't mind if you tell people how we are doing."

8. *Case:* **A 13-year-old patient's mother doesn't want us to tell her daughter that another patient with whom she had become friends has died. I know the patient will ask about her friend at some point. How should I respond?**

There is no confidentiality issue in this instance because deaths are matter of public record. For a number of reasons, it is important to meet with the parents and encourage a proactive and supportive disclosure of the friend's death. Offer ways to share the information and the option of having staff present. Discuss the mother's specific concerns about telling her daughter and suggest counter measures.

A harm may result if the child learns of the death through another patient without the supportive presence of a parent and/or a professional. Although many believe we don't have an absolute duty to always tell the truth, most would say we have an obligation not to lie. Some forms of deception (including withholding of information) are viewed as morally acceptable in some circumstances but this moral distinction may not be appreciated by the child. Well-intended withholding of information may generate distrust of parents and professionals with long-term consequences.

Generally speaking, the parent's decisions should be honored, even it creates some difficulty for the staff but in this instance, there are so many supports for telling the child the truth, it is morally permissible for the professional's principles to carry more weight in the end. If the mother remains unmoved despite efforts to counsel her to proactively inform the child, we need to respect this but be clear that we cannot lie if directly asked if the friend has died. Ask the mother if she would like you to delay answering until she can be present (if it seems feasible at the time) and offer the services of a social worker, child life specialist, or chaplain, if desired.

9. *Case:* **An 8-year-old child, whose parents are Jehovah's Witnesses, is adamant that she does not want blood during her surgery even if it means dying without it. She can tell me why blood administration is against her religion. Shouldn't we accept her wishes in this case?**

   There are a number of reasons why we should not honor her wish if it comes down to a matter of dying without the blood.

   - Her religion is not freely chosen at this stage of her life.

   - She is still in the early stages of cognitive, moral, and faith-based development (concrete operations, early conventional, and mythic-literal, respectively). Competence for making informed decisions of this serious nature does not fully exist.

   - Although her concept of death is maturing, it is likely that she does not have a fully developed adult concept, which generally occurs in early adolescence—ages 12–14.

   - Many adults who were raised in the religion of their parents later change religious affiliations. There is a chance this child's beliefs may change as a competent adult.

   - Even those who do retain key elements of the religion of their parents do not always subscribe to all tenets of the faith (e.g., many who consider themselves Catholic use artificial birth control).

   - The "best interest" and the "reasonable person" standards would favor blood administration given the disproportional burdens and benefits.

   Take the wishes of the child and family very seriously and make every effort to avoid the need for blood. If the hospital doesn't have a "bloodless medicine and surgery program," encourage physicians to contact one that does for guidance. If blood must be given (with court order), encourage involvement of church elders and, if the family desires, offer psychological counseling as needed. It is not true that the child who has received blood will be shunned by the religious community or made to feel "contaminated."

10. *Case:* **I made a mistake earlier today and gave a preschool child a double dose of an oral antibiotic. It did not and will not cause any harm to the child. I reported the mistake to the physician and the Clinical Manager. Do I tell the parents I made a mistake?**

A great deal of professional and public attention has been given to the prevalence and consequences of medical errors. There are pros and cons to disclosing a medical error that does not have any medical consequences for the child.

In this particular scenario, it is ethically permissible (neither obligatory nor forbidden) to withhold information regarding the error from the parents because:

- There is no direct harm to the patient.

- The error was reported to the physician (who could assess likelihood of harm and intervene if necessary).

- The error was reported to the manager who could address systems issues and the nurse's need for education/ monitoring.

- It cannot be known in advance whether telling will increase or decrease parental anxiety/trust.

11. *Case:* **As a male nurse in a pediatric setting I am concerned about the possibility that adolescent girls or boys (or their parents) may misconstrue sensitive exams or procedures as inappropriate heterosexual or homosexual advances. Should I just make sure I am not assigned to teenage patients?**

In our society, female nurses still tend to be the norm but the gender of the nurse is probably much less of an issue than one might think. Legitimate interventions on the part of female nurses may just as easily be viewed by their male or female patients as heterosexual or homosexual advances. Most patients have had experiences with male physicians without problem. Younger children are just as vulnerable as adolescent patients, if not even more so in some respects, to abuse of adult authority via inappropriate sexual advances.

If the patient does seem to be uncomfortable, simply say, "Sometimes kids your age are a little embarrassed about this part of the (exam or treatment), so we will get through it as quickly as possible." Provide appropriate draping, be prepared to use distraction, and ask the patient if he/she can think of anything that would make the exam/ procedure easier.

It is essential that both male and female nurses take the precaution of having a colleague or family member present during sensitive exams or treatments. Be aware that some cultures and religions may have prohibitions against care being provided by members of the opposite sex, and we should accommodate them when we can, but we should never promise what our resources may not permit us to deliver or what becomes unfairly burdensome to other staff.

12. *Case:* **A 15-year-old with a progressive and eventually fatal neuromuscular disorder has just become wheelchair-bound and is beginning to experience enough difficulty chewing and swallowing that his diet has been restricted to soft and pureed foods out of concern over aspiration. Eating has long been one of his primary pleasures and he doesn't like being different from other kids his age. We get into daily battles with him over food (he sometimes steals food from other patients' trays or has friends sneak in food items). Should we just give in and let him eat if he wants to chance the consequences?**

Truthfully, there is only so much control we are capable of exercising over his food intake if he is determined to sneak foods he should not eat. We don't want our relationship with this young man to be an adversarial one, but we also cannot give up entirely. Consider the following in your efforts to preserve both safety and quality of life:

- Hold a conference with patient and family to discuss basis of dietary restrictions and potential consequences for ignoring them. Assess the patient's ability to understand and personalize the information in a meaningful way. Assess the level of family support.

- Ensure that pureed vegetables and meats can be eaten in private and save public eating situations for such "normal" items as ice cream, pudding, yogurt, milk shakes, or chocolate bars.

- Find new activities and diversions that do not center around eating.

- Don't minimize the loss of the ability to eat normally— some counseling may be helpful.

- Consider setting up a contract with penalties and rewards.

- When facing a "battle" circumstance over contraband food, reiterate concern over the potential risks and the patient's well-being. Sympathize with the difficult choice he has to make and express confidence in his ability to make a good decision. Admit that control over the situation is largely his. Let him know that if he decides to eat the forbidden food, you will make note of it for his physician and his parents and if he chokes or aspirates, you will do your best to help him.

13. *Case:* **I am concerned about parents who don't evidence "caring" for their hospitalized child. If they room in, they stay up late at night, sleep in most of the morning, and watch soap operas all afternoon. They pay more attention to other children than their own. They sometimes leave shortly after admission, not to be seen or heard from for days. They interfere with our routine and want nurses to take total care of the child even when they are present. Should we hold them more accountable? Isn't this neglect?**

The ideal may be a fully present, fully focused, and fully involved parent who recognizes a child's need for a consistent and balanced routine. Parents who fall short in some or even many respects are not necessarily neglectful. The parent who "dumps" the child and doesn't return for 2 days may have other children at home or a job he will lose if he misses one more day of work. This may be a survival strategy rather than neglect. To the extent that the parent's absence or inattention interferes with the ability to deliver care, we should hold parents accountable. Those who won't be accountable may qualify as neglectful, although that determination requires careful and comprehensive assessment.

It helps to be clear during the admission process about hospital routines and expectations of parental availability and involvement. It is also important to negotiate alternatives when possible. Modeling of more attentive, child-focused behaviors may also have some impact but changing/improving parenting practices is not generally the primary aim of an inpatient stay and is often not practical.

14. **Case: A 6-year-old patient with chronic illness requires repeat admissions. Her single mother cannot visit often given her job, the needs of her other children, and the long drive from their hometown. Some of the nurses bring in gifts for this child or give her special floor privileges, and one of the single nurses comes in off duty to spend time with her on weekends. Is this justified in view of the unavailability of the child's mother?**

This scenario raises several issues specific to therapeutic relationships and professional boundaries. Transference and counter transference, enmeshment, fairness, staff splitting, and even legal liability are all pertinent considerations. It could be argued that it isn't "just" to do for one patient what you wouldn't/couldn't require that all nurses do for all patients under the same circumstances. Intended or not, the actions described may promote a "good nurse" [brings in gifts] versus "bad nurse" [doesn't bring in gifts] distinction. This erroneous distinction may simply exist in the mind of the patients or it may be perceived by the nurses as well, pressuring them to feel they must spend their money on gifts for their patients. Off-duty visiting raises concern over the ability of the involved nurses to achieve the desirable goal of establishing a healthy separation/balance between their personal and professional lives. Finally, it is not necessarily safe to assume the parent would approve of the gift-giving or extra visits. Some seemingly routine/innocent gifts may be offensive to the parent (for religious reasons, many parents would object to their children being given copies of the very popular Harry Potter books, for example). While some parents of limited means may be grateful that the staff have provided gifts or are visiting on their off-duty time, others may worry that these actions diminish the parents in the eyes of their children.

The following recommendations may be helpful in preventing or dealing with professional boundary violations.

- The hospital can set up a "special visitors" program for children whose families can't be present and staff may make arrangements for music and art therapy and Child Life interventions if resources are available.

- Ask for donations of pre-paid phone cards so that children separated from families may call home frequently.

- Establish policies about gift giving: limited to explicit occasions, limited in number, distributed from Child Life or Social Work or other hospital staff rather than given by individual staff.

- Establish policies about staff interactions with patients other than during delivery of care while on duty.

- Provide periodic educational offerings regarding therapeutic relations and professional boundaries.

15. *Case:* **We have a possible case of Munchausen's Syndrome by Proxy (MSBP) ("parent-induced illness" or "factitious illness by proxy") and the physicians are going to order surreptitious videotaping. I am very uncomfortable about this. Isn't this an unethical intrusion?**

Surreptitious videotaping is a very intrusive intervention as the patient, the family, many staff, and all visitors will be videotaped without their knowledge and consent. MSBP is a serious condition that is difficult to diagnose, results in unnecessary diagnostic tests, medical and surgical interventions and hospitalizations, and sometimes, lifelong physical or psychological disability or death. The financial cost is staggering and healthcare professionals become unwitting accomplices of the perpetrators of this child abuse.

The primary purpose of videotaping is making a diagnosis, not solving a crime; however, because a crime is involved, videotaping should be undertaken in a way that meets requirements for preserving the chain of evidence. Because of their nature, some MSBP cases can be diagnosed by other means (e.g., blood typing that demonstrates the blood in the diaper did not come from the baby or toxicology screens that reveal the presence of drugs). Other cases (such as smothering) are best diagnosed by videotaping. Hospitals wishing to use surreptitious videotaping should have policies that address the following:

- Circumstances that warrant videotaping
- Diagnostic measures that should be exhausted prior to resorting to video
- Key players to be involved in the decision making and those who must be notified once the decision has been made (e.g., administration, legal department)
- Point at which public children's services agency should be notified given the suspicion of abuse
- Process involved in assuring maintenance of chain of evidence
- Continuous, live, off-site monitoring of the videotaping versus simply viewing select sections of video upon the alleged occurrence of an "event"
- Authorization of video viewing
- Approach to family once the diagnosis is made. What resources need to be in place?
- Documentation standards (keep in mind, parents may access the medical record at any point)
- Role of the hospital's Child Protection Team and/or the Ethics Committee

16. *Case:* **We have a family visiting from the Middle East in order to obtain medical care for their child. The father has forbidden some medical interventions that could make a difference in the quality of his daughter's life and that are considered fairly routine in our country. I know the mother really wants the proce-**

dures to be undertaken but in her country the father makes all the decisions. We strongly suspect that the father would consent to the procedures if the child were a boy. Would it be wrong for me to speak out as an advocate for the child and her mother?

The culture of the patient/family has a profound influence on decision making and should be accorded significant respect. There are circumstances where the family's cultural beliefs should not be permitted to dictate care but there must be serious overriding concerns and the burden of proof should fall to the medical team.

It would be ethically permissible (perhaps even obligatory) to make a concerted effort to persuade the father to agree to the procedures. A care conference might be a helpful intervention and an ethics consultation with the family is another avenue for pursuit. Consider involving a member of the clergy of the family's faith if this resource is available and family is open to it. In this case, if the father remains adamant, it would not be acceptable to override his decision for the following reasons:

- The child is receiving quality medical care and will be leaving in an improved state of health. Failure to undertake the additional interventions will not compromise the success of the medical care they sought.

- We are not talking about life and death interventions but quality of life and we are not risking a quality of life that is not worth living if the additional procedures are not performed.

- We are being limited in our ability to provide benefit or "do good" but we are not being asked to do harm.

- The family comes from and will return to a culture that is supportive of the differential valuation and treatment of women, vests the male parent with decision-making authority, and may put a different premium on quality of life issues.

17. *Case:* **A 16-year-old patient went to the cafeteria with some visiting friends. When he came back, he smelled of alcohol. I confronted him and he admitted his friends sneaked him some beer. They usually**

have a few beers on weekends, and his parents are unaware that he drinks. He has begged me not to tell. What is my obligation?

Against Telling

- Although he is not legally or functionally a fully autonomous person, he does have some rights to privacy and confidentiality and there are some legal protections specific to substance use/treatment and adolescents.

- He does not appear intoxicated or otherwise harmed (a physician should determine whether the beer intake could negatively affect medical condition or treatment).

- "Telling" sometimes jeopardizes parent/child relationships and may put some teens at risk of abusive retaliation.

- Disclosing may generate distrust for the healthcare team and lessen the likelihood that the patient will continue to confide truthfully when it is critical to care decisions or that he will comply with medical care.

In Favor of Telling

- He and his friends are not of legal drinking age and are stealing or being illegally supplied with alcohol. Parents have a responsibility to keep him safe and instill better values but are handicapped without the information.

- The drinking occurred on hospital premises while hospital staff was responsible for the well-being of the patient.

- The observations and assessment of the patient's condition do need to be documented in the medical record if only for liability reasons. Most parents don't ask to review medical records but they do have the right to do so and could find out anyway.

- Although he doesn't seem impaired now, he and his friends may have true problems with alcohol (and other substances for which alcohol is the gateway "drug"). Failure to tell may be a missed opportunity for parents to intervene early.

A responsible approach to this controversial dilemma should include the following:

- Skilled substance abuse assessment (Social Worker, Clinical Nurse Specialist, Physician) and assessment of social situation (in particular, risks associated with telling parents)

- Firmly encourage the teen to tell (or allow the team to tell) parents of the incident. Provide the reasons for doing so and advise him that parents may find out anyway if they review the medical record. Offer to rehearse the telling and to discuss how to manage any fallout feared by the patient.

- Absent an assessment suggestive of substance abuse or potential impact on current medical condition and treatment, if patient steadfastly refuses parental notification, it is morally permissible (some would say morally obligatory) to respect his confidentiality. However, it is important to provide the teen with information about substance use and abuse and drug/alcohol treatment referral information. He should also be told that there is to be no further alcohol consumption or his parents will be informed. You might consider restriction to the floor and supervision of visiting from a risk management perspective.

18. *Case:* **A 14-year-old patient's parents are divorced and his mother is planning to remarry in a few months. My patient says he doesn't like his future stepfather and doesn't want him to visit or to be given information by any members of the healthcare team. His mother and her boyfriend are insisting otherwise. The biological father is not involved. Is it right to honor the patient's request?**

Though not legally or functionally autonomous, a 14-year-old does have the right to some privacy and confidentiality, even with respect to biologic/custodial parents. The mother's boyfriend has an interest but no legal standing and little or no moral standing. There is no way to know with certainty that he and the mother will end up married.

Potential harms if teen's wishes are respected are:

- Strain on present and (possibly long-term) relationship between mother and child (particularly if mother decides to share information with boyfriend anyway).

- Decreased likelihood of positive family dynamics should the marriage take place.

- Strained relationship between parent and healthcare team.

- If teen has significant ongoing healthcare needs, this is a lost opportunity for teaching/preparation of future stepfather.

Potential harms if teen's wishes are not respected are:

- Teen's experience of privacy violation (even more grievous if the marriage never occurs).

- Decreased trust in and cooperation with medical team on the part of the patient.

- Possibly some legal liability for the hospital (violation of HIPAA).

Prior to honoring the patient's request, there should be some discussion with him. He should also understand that his mother might choose to share the information that the staff withholds. There should be an attempt to get the mother to understand and respect the patient's requests and an attempt to have the two negotiate a mutually satisfying outcome. If negotiations fail, the teen's privacy and confidentiality interests should prevail. A strong recommendation should be made for both individual and family counseling prior to committing fully to the marriage.

19. **Case: The nursing staff members have a lot of angry feelings toward a mother whose husband was abusing her 4-year-old daughter over quite some period of time. The father is in jail and they believe the mother should be too, or at the very least, she should not be allowed to visit. What is our responsibility toward this mother who failed to protect her child?**

The making of informed, analytical, and compassionate judgments is a nursing responsibility, but prejudice and judgmentalism have no place. Though nurses sometimes assume some of the responsibilities particular to the role of a social worker or even a detective, determinations about custody, visitation, and criminal complicity do not fall to the nursing staff. This is a known case of abuse that is being investigated by the police and the public children's services agency. The role of the nurse is to address the child's medical and emotional needs and provide objective observations investigating agents may find useful in making their determinations. This mother may be just as much a victim (of domestic violence) as the child. Depriving the child of contact with the mother may be another victimization of the child.

Nurses must, as professionals, partner with this parent as they would with any other unless there is clear, objective evidence of abuse or neglect on her part. Staff may need some opportunities to vent their emotions. An inservice about the family dynamics of abuse and domestic violence may be helpful. The ability to function compassionately and effectively in this challenging circumstance is a reflection of the "art" of professional nursing.

20. *Case:* **A child with multiple handicaps who is severely mentally compromised spends all his time here in the hospital or in a chronic care facility. His parents rarely visit in either location. Some serious medical decisions have to be made and staff disagrees with the parents' choices. Staff members believe they know the child far better and that they are the ones who have truly "parented" this child. Is it ethical to leave the decision making to the parents in this instance?**

By default, it is the right and responsibility of parents to make healthcare decisions on behalf of their children. Although parents have delegated the care of their child to people they believe are in a better position to address his complex healthcare needs and although they seldom visit, that does not mean they have forsaken their role or that they are unfit or incompetent. It may be true that some staff "know" the child more intimately than he/she knows the parents but that does not mean the parents are not making good faith decisions in what they believe to be the best interests of the child.

A care conference involving representatives from all disciplines within the care team, the family, and anyone they believe would be of support to them (relatives, clergy, family physician, etc.) is a good preliminary step. This may be all that is needed to assuage staff concerns or persuade parents to change their minds. A next step, if either the team or the parents desire, would be an ethics consultation. If resolution is not achieved and the healthcare team still feels that decisions are being made that are not in the best interest of the child, an appeal can be made to the public children's services agency or a request can be made for court-ordered care. These are advocacy measures on behalf of the child but at the same time are adversarial moves with respect to the parents.

What would suggest that the adversarial approach is necessary?

- Violations of respect for the dignity of the child
- Violations of the duty to do good and avoid harm (harmful consequences—burdens clearly outweigh the benefits)
- Justice violations (failure to provide the same care one could justify providing all others in morally relevant circumstances)
- Clear indications that parents are in some way incompetent or acting out of a conflict of interest

RESOURCES

American Academy of Bioethics, Bioethics Policy. http://www.aap.org/visit/Bio ethicsPolicy.htm

Beauchamp, T. L., & Childress, J. R. (2001). *Principles of biomedical ethics.* New York: Oxford University Press.

Bioethics.net. http://www.bioethics.net/

Garrett, M. T., Baillie, H. W., & Garrett, R. M. (2000). *Health care ethics: Principles & problems.* Englewood Cliffs, NJ: Prentice Hall.

Initiative for Pediatric Palliative Care. http://www.ippcweb.org

PedsCCM: The Pediatric Critical Care Website (ethics bibliography). http://peds ccm.wustl.edu/File-cabinet/file_cab_section2.html

Pence, G. F. (2004). *Classic cases in medical ethics.* Boston: McGraw Hill.

Thomas, R. M. (1997). *Moral developmental theories—Secular and religious: A comparative study* . Westport, CT: Greenwood Press.

Veatch, R. M. (2003). *The basics of bioethics.* Englewood Cliffs, NJ: Prentice Hall.

Part 3

Ethical Issues With Vulnerable Patients

Nurses' own biases and judgments come to the forefront with the patients in these groups who are viewed as vulnerable. We are challenged to remember that the ANA (2001) *Code* states, "The nurse respects the worth, dignity and rights of all human beings irrespective of the nature of the health problems" (p. 7). Protecting the rights of patients with psychiatric illness requires vigilance; many of the questions speak to this responsibility. Since the first cases of Human Immunodeficiency Virus, diagnosed in 1981, many myths and ethical questions regarding its transmission have flooded the media. The chapter authors in part 3 work daily with these patients and, therefore, provide insight into how to respond to the questions. Lack of adherence with treatment, medication, and diet regimen is often frustrating to nurses. These chapters will address some of the questions you have asked about these behaviors. As baby boomers age, they also become interested in the plight of the elderly in nursing homes. The authors will address the host of ethical issues in long-term care.

Chapter 10

Psychiatric Patients and Ethical Issues

Deborah Antai-Otong

1. How much and what type of information is appropriate to disclose to patients?

It is important for you to understand that establishing and maintaining a healthy and therapeutic relationship requires an understanding of your role. Your role in a therapeutic relationship is a nurse provider and not "friend." Facilitating healthy interpersonal relationship begins with defining and maintaining healthy boundaries between you and patients.

Demanding patients are the most challenging because they sometimes insist that the nurse disclose personal information to restore equality or demonstrate the nurse's commitment to the patient and treatment. It may be helpful to discuss your concerns with an experienced advanced practice psychiatric nurse or mental health professional. Any of the following could create or contribute to boundary problems: need to be seen as indispensable; need for intimacy; unsatisfied personal life; over-identification with patient (e.g., same age, ethnicity, personal characteristics); life insecure because of physical or psychological distress; burnout, lack of knowledge about boundaries; and unhealthy need to be responsible for others.

Considerations for self-disclosure must be carefully scrutinized to maintain healthy boundaries between yourself and patients. Boundaries often depict the edge of professional behavior and are influenced by the therapeutic contract, consent, and context of the relationship. Boundary violations are generally destructive and are usually exploitive of patient needs (e.g., financial, dependency, control). You must learn how to recognize potential harmful areas as risk factors that result in inappropriate self-disclosure.

2. What is the most appropriate response to a patient who asks me for a date?

Boundaries define the expected and accepted psychological and social distance between nurses and their patients. Patients asking you for a date are blurring the boundaries in the nurse-patient relationship. The request could be a result of transference, manipulation, or a genuine affectionate request. However, whatever the reason, the nurse has the ethical responsibility to define the relationship as therapeutic only.

Maintain your composure, respond assertively, and assess the patient's response to your comments. An example of an appropriate response is, "I value our nurse-patient relationship. My role is that of providing medications and monitoring your response to treatment and not that of a person you could take on a date."

3. What criteria are generally used to determine if a patient needs to be involuntarily committed?

The criteria for involuntary commitment vary from state to state. You need to determine the state laws that govern involuntary commitment. Normally, patients who are involuntarily committed exhibit behaviors and symptoms that pose a threat to self and/or others. This may involve acute and severe symptoms of mental illness, drug intoxication/withdrawal, and overt threats to kill self/others.

4. When a patient tells me that he plans to kill someone, what is my ethical responsibility?

It was concluded in *Tarasoff v. Regents of the University of California* (1974) "that when a doctor or psychotherapist, in the exercise of his professional skill and knowledge, determines or should determine, that a warning is essential to avert danger arising from the medical or psychological condition of his [sic] patient, he insures [sic] a legal obligation to give that warning." The court concluded that "the protective privilege ends where the public peril begins." Therefore, when a patient presents a serious danger of violence to another, the nurse incurs an obligation to use reasonable care to protect the intended victim. The foreseeability is determined by three factors: (1) a history of violence; (2) a threat to a named or clearly identifiable victim; (3) a plausible motive. If at least two of the three factors are present, courts have generally found a duty to warn. Therefore, your ethical responsibility is to forewarn the identified potential victim.

If the patient calls via phone, efforts to stay in contact are crucial, especially if the police attempt to trace the call. Inquiring about reasons for present thoughts of harm, means, intent, and past gestures is crucial because these factors help determine the level of lethality. Facilities need to be proactive in addressing this issue by establishing policies that address these calls.

5. What safeguards are included in the Americans With Disabilities Act (ADA) for persons with psychiatric and substance-related disorders?

The ADA is designed to integrate persons with disabilities fully into the mainstream of American life. The Act explicitly includes persons with mental disabilities and prohibits discrimination in employment and public accommodation.

Reasonable accommodations may include job-restructuring, acquisition of equipment and devices, and policy changes, such as nurses not giving opioids to patient without supervision. In the ADA definition, "an individual with disability" does not include an individual who is currently engaging in illegal use of drugs or has a gambling addiction. For the purpose of this Act, a qualified individual with a disability refers to an individual who with or without reasonable accommodation can perform the essential functions of the employed position.

6. What questions are helpful in assessing a patient's level of danger to self and/or others?

Ask the patient about recent stressors including recent/significant losses or reasons for wanting to kill self.

A thorough suicidal assessment includes the following:

1. Ask the patient if he/she has thoughts of killing self. If yes . . .

2. What is your plan? If yes . . .

3. Do you have the means? If yes . . .

4. What has stopped you from acting on the thoughts?

5. What types of stressors are you experiencing that have led you to considering suicide at this time?

6. Have you tried to kill yourself in the past? If yes . . .

7. What did you do? What type of treatment did you receive? What was going on in your life at the time(s)?

Initially, it is imperative for you to determine if the patient has a plan, but it is equally important to assess present stressors and verify if there is a past history of suicide. A past history of suicide is the greatest predictor of present and future acts and indicates the patient's coping patterns.

7. *Case:* **A patient with schizophrenia has been admitted to the unit exhibiting acute psychotic symptoms, and one of the research assistants asks him to sign an informed consent to participate in a new drug study. What is my responsibility in ensuring this patient's rights?**

The first question is "does the patient have the capacity to understand and decide?" If this individual is exhibiting acute psychotic symptoms, one would conclude that the patient does not have the capacity and could not commit on a voluntary basis to participate in this study. The voluntary consent of a human subject is absolutely necessary. This means that the person involved should have legal capacity to consent and should be able to exert free power of choice without duress. The patient's decisional capacity is the basis of informed consent and includes the patient's ability to comprehend and logically process information as well as the ability to communicate the decision.

Experts in the field of informed consent propose a process of tripartite consent for research in schizophrenia, which always requires a more exacting standard of disclosure than treatment. This process calls for a duty to protect vulnerable individuals and provide meaningful oversight by three objective professionals with the responsibility, expertise, and authority to facilitate the prospective participants' understanding of consent disclosures.

8. *Case:* A patient with schizophrenia is seen during a home visit and complains of concerns about her medication because a family member told her that her medication was dangerous and that if she does not stop taking it she will end up in a wheelchair. This patient has a history of nonadherence to treatment and currently takes a haloperidol D. What is the most appropriate response to this patient?

Most neuroleptic antipsychotic agents, particularly conventional agents, such as haloperidol, are more likely to produce movement disorders, including tardive dyskinesia as compared to novel agents (e.g., clozapine, quetiapine). Various screening tools, such as the Abnormal Involuntary Movement Scale (AIMS) help you assess early signs of tardive dyskinesia (e.g., excessive blinking, frowning, mouth movements), an irreversible and disabling movement disorder.

An appropriate response to a concerned patient can include, "I understand your concerns about your medication. Let's review the benefits of taking this medication and potential side effects. I also want to ask you a few questions to assess how you are responding to your medication."

9. **What is the rationale for giving a patient medication (chemical restraints) against his/her will?**

The decision to medicate against a person will is guided by state mental health codes. A common rationale is that the patient is a danger to self and others and is being evaluated under a 72-hour emergency order of protective custody. Restraints of any kind are only used when patients are so dangerous they cannot be controlled in any other way. Chemical restraints indicate a psychiatric emergency and, therefore, must be used in combination with constant monitoring. In the case of a patient withdrawing from alcohol, it is best to prevent DTs by giving benzodiazepine early. It is unethical to use as punishment or for the convenience of the staff.

10. *Case:* During a home visit I noticed that a family member had overmedicated a patient who has a developmental disorder. What is my ethical responsibility?

It is important to determine if overdosing occurred for convenience, lack of knowledge on the family member's part, or the patient is having an adverse response and dosage needs to be lowered. Initially, assess the patient's mental and physical status. Express your concerns about the patient's mental and physical state and if assessment warrants, call for immediate medical attention via 911. Inquire about the patient's current medication, dose, and if he/she has responded this way in the past. Once the patient is medically stable, report your findings to the appropriate agency for further medical evaluation and potential abuse. Also assess the family member's understanding and knowledge about the medication, dosage, and potential side effects, and provide health education.

11. **Case: A homosexual couple comes into the office seeking psychotherapy to deal with relationship problems. The nurse therapist has strong objections to homosexual behavior and believes that he cannot deal with this couple because of lack of objectivity or acceptance of the couple's behavior. What is the most appropriate way to handle these feelings and situation?**

In 1973, homosexuality was eliminated as a diagnostic category by the American Psychiatric Association and removed from the *DSM* in 1980. Sexual orientation alone is not to be regarded as a disorder. This change reflects a change in understanding homosexuality, which is now considered to be a variant of human sexuality, not a pathological disorder. The presence of homosexuality does not appear to be a matter of choice. Therefore, as a nurse you need to seek professional supervision to gain a greater understanding of homosexuality as a natural expression of a human's sexual nature as is heterosexuality.

Acknowledging negative responses is important, but it is also imperative to understand that you will meet patients whose values differ from yours. In order to reduce the harm of transferring the care to another therapist, use the interdisciplinary team to help you resolve your strong reactions. To be an effective therapist you need to learn how to work with patients whose values and beliefs differ from yours.

12. *Case:* **An adolescent is brought into the emergency room complaining of suicidal thoughts and during the course of your evaluation, you inquire about access to weapons. His parents state that their guns are locked up and that their son does not have a key. What steps do you need to take to ensure the youth's safety?**

    Suicide is the third leading cause of death in the 15- to 24-year-old age group; therefore, the threat must be taken seriously. The absence of a strong social support system, history of impulsive behavior, and a suicidal plan are indications for hospitalization. I would question the parents' support and understanding about the dangerousness of access to guns if they refuse to remove the guns from the home.

    Convey your concerns about the adolescent's safety and the importance of reducing the availability of firearms by removing them from the home. If the parents opt to leave them in the home, it is imperative to document the conversation about firearms with the parents and their choice to keep weapons in the home. If the parents express concerns about removing weapons from the home or where to store them, encourage them to contact the local police department for assistance.

13. *Case:* **A 14-year-old patient reveals that she is sexually active and is taking birth control pills without her parents' consent. She states that her parents are "real religious" and she is afraid they will get upset because she usually shares "everything with them." What is the most appropriate way to handle this information and what part should you share with the parents?**

    A challenge for psychiatric nurses is what to share with parents about their adolescents. Sometimes we are torn between what the parent should know versus what they must know. Establishing trust with an adolescent is very difficult because, in general, they do not trust adults. When working with adolescents it is crucial to discuss confidentiality and explicate circumstances where it cannot be maintained (e.g., danger to self or others).

You can convey support by using the following comments: "I know that discussing sexual matters with your parents is difficult. However, since you have a close relationship with them they may be more understanding than you think." If the adolescent opts to discuss this matter with her parents, let her know that you are available to meet with them. Regardless of the adolescent's decision, you must impart understanding and empathy.

14. **Case: Mr. Jones is a 65-year-old who is brought to the emergency department with severe abdominal pain. He also has a history of severe depression and has been off his antidepressant for several months. The ED physician suspects acute appendicitis. He refuses to sign the consent form because he does not trust anyone and fears evil things will happen while he is under anesthesia. The physician states that the patient is incompetent. How does his depression affect competency?**

Declaring someone incompetent is a legal process. A related, but different term is "capacity," which is considered a functional matter that refers to specific deficits. This patient may be able to handle his financial matters, but may be unable to make a decision as to whether to have surgery for acute appendicitis. Psychological incapacity can result from a temporary or permanent deficit in neurobiological process such as psychosis or severe depression.

Depressed patients often feel hopeless, selectively perceive negative information, and frequently conclude that interventions will not succeed. Mild to moderate depression has little predictive value in determining the preferences toward life-sustaining treatment. However, in patients who are severely depressed, recovery from depression is associated with increased desire for life-saving medical therapy. In general, life-sustaining treatment should not be withheld until efforts have been made to reverse the depression. Therefore, a psychiatric consult is warranted in this case.

15. *Case:* You overhear one of your co-workers making racial statements about a patient who is in seclusion. Specifically, he states, "we need to keep him medicated because of his race." What is the most appropriate way to handle this situation?

    None of us likes to be on the receiving end of prejudice, but most of us have been. Prejudice implies a preconceived and unreasonable judgment or opinion, usually an unfavorable one marked by suspicion, fear, intolerance, and hatred. Prejudice is considered irrational because it is not based on facts; the opinion is often held despite facts. When we support prejudice, either by overt action or by condoning through our silence, we add to the injury or harm resulting from the judgment/action of others.

    Approach the staff member in an assertive manner and express your concerns about the comments. For instance, "it really concerns me that you are making unproven comments about this patient." Depending upon her response, you may have an opportunity to educate her about cultural and ethnic issues concerning mental health and treatment strategies. It is also important to stress how the staff person's comments and biases may interfere with accurately assessing the patient's symptoms and preferences and developing appropriate treatment planning.

16. *Case:* A homeless patient comes into the outpatient community center and reports that someone stole his wallet and he needs a pack of cigarettes to calm his "nerves." He asks you for money to buy cigarettes. How would you respond to this patient?

    State "I am sorry to hear about your situation, but I am unwilling to give you money for cigarettes. What else can I help you with?" Determine if he will let you have him evaluated for a housing program for the chronically mentally ill. Many homeless suffer from schizophrenia or schizoaffective disorder, which may be the origin of the story of the lost wallet. If he refuses evaluation or the offer of shelter, see what you can do to link him to appropriate community mental health resources.

17. *Case:* **A patient is brought to the psychiatric triage unit with an overdose of an opiate and is on life support. His neighbor calls and states that he knows that he has overdosed and wants to get an update on his condition so he can share it with his family. How much, if any, information is confidential under these circumstances?**

Long-term premises of nursing ethics binds nurses to hold secret all information given by the patient. A group that is within the circle of confidentiality shares information without getting the patient's permission. Parties outside the circle would include the neighbor.

HIPAA regulations define who can share what information with whom and what sort of approval must be secured prior to sharing the information. Oftentimes, neighbors are truly concerned about their neighbors' well-being, particularly under these circumstances. However, according to HIPAA regulations, you cannot share any information with a neighbor concerning this patient's condition. If you have not made contact with the family, ask the neighbor to put you in touch with the family. Inform him that the family will then be the avenue for information on the patient.

18. *Case:* **A patient calls in on the crisis hotline threatening to kill himself and his family because his wife has asked for a divorce. What are some crucial questions to ask when you are on a hotline that enable you to assess further this patient's level of danger to self and others?**

Having recently experienced a significant loss implies increased risk. Other high-risk criteria include being a male over 45 years of age who is widowed or divorced, is unemployed, and has conflictual interpersonal relationships. Other factors include a sense of hopelessness, previous attempts, chronic illness, and substance abuse. If his family is unresponsive to his pain, he has the lethal means, and is socially isolated, he could require hospitalization.

Acknowledge and convey empathy about his level of distress and inquire about his location, telephone number and whether he has a weapon, past history of suicide, psychiatric or substance-related problems. Ask him to agree to a no-suicide or no-harm contract. If the patient cannot make an agreement to call when he/she becomes uncertain about the ability to control suicidal impulses, then hospitalization is needed.

19. *Case:* **A couple brings in their 10-year-old child who is currently taking an atypical neuroleptic agent for conduct disorder. They are expressing delight in the youth's behavior over the past few months since he began taking this medication. You notice that the child has excessive frowning, grimacing, mouth movements, and a slow gait. What is the most appropriate response to the parents and how much should you discuss about the child's present demeanor and behavior with them?**

Focus your response on further assessment with comments such as, "I can see that you are pleased about your son's progress. However, I am concerned about his facial movements. How long has your son been on this medication, what is his current dose, and how long has he had these symptoms?" Inquire about their understanding of these side effects of the neuroleptic. Ask "when was the last time he saw the provider who wrote the prescription?" Express concerns about these symptoms and encourage them to follow up with the provider as soon as possible to evaluate them.

20. *Case:* **A local police officer accompanies Mr. M to the ER with a mental illness warrant and reports that he has been threatening to stab his youngest sibling. An order has been written to give him an injection of haloperidol. He refuses the medication. What are your ethical responsibilities in complying with his right in refusing this medication?**

Although the definition of mental illness warrant varies from state to state, the general meaning involves being able to administer medication involuntarily when there is clinical evidence that the patient's psychiatric symptoms pose a danger to self and/or others. In addition, these laws usually stipulate that under a mental health warrant the medication can be administered.

For example, a patient's mother calls 911 after the patient threatened to stab her, because "the voices told him that she was the devil." The patient's history reveals that he has been off his neuroleptic medication for several weeks and that his recurrent psychosis was an imminent danger to his mother. The nurse may not forcibly administer medication unless the patient is deemed an imminent danger to self or others. If the nurse refuses to administer medication under the auspices of a mental health warrant, owing to patient's refusal, and he hurts himself or others, the nurse's actions will be reviewed by the hospital and possible court to determine if the incident was preventable.

RESOURCES

Antai-Otong, D. (2004). *Psychiatric emergencies*. Eau Claire, WI: Professional Education Systems Institute, LLC.

Chen, D. T., Miller, F. G., & Rosenstein, D. L. (2002). Enrolling decisionally impaired adults in clinical research. *Medical Care, 40*, V20–29.

Hendricks, A. L., & Barloon, L. F. (2003). Legal and ethical considerations. In D. Antai-Otong (Ed.), *Psychiatric nursing: Biological and behavioral concepts* (pp. 167–191). Clifton Park, NY: Delmar Thomson Learning.

Interim-Research Involving Individuals With Questionable Capacity to Consent: Points to Consider. http://grants.nih.gov/grants/policy/questionablecapacity.htm

Issues to Consider in Intervention Research With Persons at High Risk for Suicidality. http://www.nimh.nih.gov/SuicideResearch/highrisksuicide.cfm

Martinez, R. (2000). A model for boundary dilemmas: Ethical decision-making in the patient-professional relationship. *Ethical Human Sciences and Services, 2*, 43–61.

National Clearing House for Alcohol and Drug Information: Legal and Ethical Issues in the Treatment of Adolescents With Substance Use Disorders. http://www.health.org/govpubs/bkd307/32k.aspx

Posever, T. A., & Chelmow, T. (2001). Informed consent for research for schizophrenia: An alternative for special studies. *IRB: A Review of Human Subjects Review, 23*(1), 10–15.

Stiles, P. G., Poythress, N. G., Hall, A., Falkenbach, D., & Williams, R. (2001). Improving understanding of research consent disclosures among persons with mental illness. *Psychiatric Services, 52*, 780–785.

Chapter 11

HIV-AIDS Patients and Ethical Issues

Diane E. Radvansky

1. What actually is HIV and how is it transmitted?

Since the first cases of the Human Immunodeficiency Virus (HIV) were diagnosed in 1981, many ethical questions regarding the transmission of the virus have arisen.

HIV is a retrovirus that is transmitted through the exchange of body fluids. These exchanges can take place by needle sharing, unprotected sexual intercourse (vaginal, rectal or anal), transmission from mother to child through breast milk, and blood transfusions. These are the tangible causes of HIV transmission. HIV is not transmitted through tears, saliva, insects, toilet seats, swimming pools, linens, dishes, utensils, or a government conspiracy.

2. How can the lack of autonomy of an individual be a cause of HIV transmission?

As nurses we encounter people in practice who are powerless either due to economic reasons or their position in society. These are the people at the greatest risk of becoming infected with HIV. They are not free to make decisions about their sexual relationships or to insist on fidelity in their partners or require their partners to use condoms. In other words, they lack autonomy to protect themselves from HIV transmission.

3. Shouldn't people who practice risky behaviors be forced to give up their individual rights in order to protect the public health?

The benefit to public health must warrant the extent of intrusion into personal liberties. This principle does not suggest that public health should be sacrificed in order to protect civil liberties, but only that an uncertain or minimal public health benefit should not be used to justify gross invasion of personal rights.

To some ill-informed people, denying individuals their right to autonomy and self-determination is a "quick fix" to prevent the transmission of HIV. People who lack knowledge of HIV transmission believe that isolating "infected" individuals from the "non-infected" community will put an end to the virus. This practice infringes on the individual's right. Mandatory testing of people who are perceived to have risky lifestyles has been another "solution" offered to curb the transmission of HIV. This practice would also be an infringement of an individual's right of self-determination.

4. Can a person with HIV be denied health and/or life insurance or a job?

Federal law (The Americans With Disabilities Act) gives individuals the right to the same insurance coverage provided to other employees if they work for an employer with 15 or more employees. Individuals with HIV cannot be singled out for special treatment. If the individuals are part of a small employee group, many states now guarantee access to small group coverage regardless of health, but in many states individuals can be excluded. In about half the states, there are high-risk pools for uninsured individuals. But there are still a few states with no options at all. In all of these circumstances, there may be a waiting period for coverage of any pre-existing conditions.

Life and disability insurance will be much more difficult. In some states, people can purchase small amounts on a "guaranteed issue" basis from special risk brokers. Most people, however, will only be able to get life and disability coverage by going to work full time as part of a large employee group.

Insurance carriers can legally deny insurance if an individual has HIV or AIDS. However, HIV positive individuals do have certain rights. An insurance company cannot test for HIV without consent. However, if an individual refuses to have an HIV test, the insurance carrier can deny him/ her insurance.

People living with the virus must be aware of their individual rights regarding employment. Fortunately, it is illegal for any employer to fire an HIV positive person because they are living with the virus. Not only is it illegal to fire these individuals, they also cannot be demoted, transferred, or denied vacation or sick time. This is true for as long as the employee is able to do his/her job. Another point of interest concerning employment: if a person living with HIV should become sick and disabled because of HIV disease, the employer must make "reasonable accommodations" for the employee so that the employee can do his/her job.

5. Why is it so important to keep the HIV diagnosis confidential?

The main reason is the fear of discrimination in the community, family, or workplace. Although there are laws to protect the rights of people living with the virus against discrimination, sometimes taking legal action is not always the answer. Not all acts of discrimination can be rectified in the court system; do you sue co-workers for not sitting with you at lunch, or family members for not inviting you to dinner, or merchants for refusing to serve you?

On the other hand, some patients who have disclosed their HIV status to their communities, families, and workplace have been received openly by those they have told they have HIV. Some patients have told me that their family suspected that they were positive but felt uncomfortable confronting them about it. Once they shared their diagnosis, they were comforted by the support they received. So as you can see, it is not an easy decision either way. Nurses should help patients weigh the pros and cons of disclosing their status.

6. If HIV testing is confidential, why are the patient's name and other identifying information used when reporting patients with AIDS to the public health department?

Currently the names of patients with AIDS are reported to the public health department but names of HIV-positive patients are not reported. Patients with AIDS are reported in order to monitor the epidemic, plan and design HIV services and prevention programs, and allocate resources.

HIV-positive individuals' names are not as yet reported in all states. There has been much controversy regarding reporting of names on HIV tests. As it stands now, patients tested for HIV can either give their "real" name or use only initials. Name reporting of HIV-positive patients is not required in order to encourage at risk individuals to be tested. At risk individuals have indicated that if their names were reported on the test application, they would not have been tested for fear of disclosure to insurance companies, employers. Until people living with the virus believe that their individual rights will be respected, they will not consent to name reporting.

There are two reasons why name reporting of HIV-positive patients is being considered. Many patients come into the outreach centers or community centers to be tested and do not provide identifying information. When the HIV test results are positive and the clients do not return to obtain their results, they are not aware of their HIV status. Therefore, clients are not receiving medical care or counseling, or taking measures to prevent the transmission of HIV.

Service allocation is the second reason name reporting of HIV-positive patients is being considered. With improved treatment of HIV, many patients do not progress to AIDS and are not being counted. Reporting HIV-positive patients enables a better count of HIV cases. Knowing this information will be helpful in providing services and prevention programs.

7. What recourse does a patient have if HIV status has been disclosed without his/her permission?

The individual can take legal action. However, the individual must be aware that by using the court system he/she may inadvertently be disclosing his/her HIV status. HIV-positive litigants have some alternatives. Some courts are allowing the litigant to file a lawsuit using a pseudonym, using just initials, or requesting the court for an order sealing the case record or for a protective order with the court.

8. What moral obligations do HIV-positive healthcare workers have to report their HIV status to their employer and to their patients?

Healthcare workers must follow the ethical principle of non-maleficence. We have the duty to act in the best interest of patients regardless of whether our own interests are harmed. That means if we are performing an exposure prone procedure the patient has the right to know our HIV status, even if this could cause harm to ourselves.

Healthcare personnel living with HIV infection have a right to continue working as healthcare providers and to be assured of confidentiality about their HIV status in all cases. The Centers for Disease Control and Prevention did not document a single case of HIV transmission from 63 HIV-infected healthcare workers to any of their more than 22,000 patients. Based on the lack of any confirmed cases, the risk of transmission of HIV from provider to patient is judged to be so small that practice restrictions do not appear warranted. Disclosing HIV status in the workplace can have some advantages, including scheduling flexibility and avoidance of exposure to opportunistic and other infections. Healthcare workers must evaluate whom they can trust with this sensitive information.

9. Do healthcare workers have the autonomy to refuse caring for HIV-positive patients if they believe their safety is at risk?

Nurses have a professional duty to treat all patients. The major concern of healthcare providers is the risk of occupational exposure to HIV. The risk of occupational HIV infection is small but is not nonexistent. The Centers for Disease Control and Prevention has determined that people with HIV may be treated safely by practicing Universal Precautions. Therefore, the Americans With Disabilities Act stated that it is illegal to refuse to treat a patient with HIV based on fear of transmission. As a guide, nurses should refer to the *Code of Ethics for Nurses* that states:

> The nurse, in all professional relationships, practices with compassion and respect for the inherent dignity, worth and uniqueness of every individual, unrestricted by consideration of social or economic status, personal attributes, or of the nature of health problems. (ANA, 2001, p. 7)

10. Why does testing a patient for HIV require an informed consent when no consent is required for other blood tests? Are there any exceptions to this informed consent?

Any person being tested for HIV cannot be tested without informed consent and pre- and posttest counseling. The pretest counseling includes information on what the test is testing, how HIV is transmitted, and assessment of the individual's risky behaviors and discussion of risk-reduction practices. Posttest counseling must be given to the person at the time he/she receives the results. Posttest counseling provides the HIV-positive individuals with referrals to medical care and psychological counseling, information about HIV and AIDS, and treatment options. Informed consent is required for this blood test because positive HIV results can have a profound impact on an individual's life.

There are two exceptions. The first exception to the law states that a person who is found guilty of rape, or who has pled guilty to a charge of rape, can be tested for HIV without his/her agreement if the victim requests it. The victim of the rape will get the test results. Another exception is that a judge can order you to be tested or to reveal your HIV status after a court hearing. First you will get a chance to present evidence about why your status should not be revealed.

11. What is my ethical responsibility as a healthcare provider to patients who have HIV and continue to have unprotected sex?

Reinforce to the patient at each health encounter that not practicing safe sex is irresponsible behavior. Suggestions are offered of various safe sex practices, such as offering a female condom to a woman whose partner refuses to use a male condom. Patients should also be aware that not only are they protecting their partners, but also themselves from resistant strains of HIV and other sexually transmitted diseases. Condoms should be easily accessible to all patients. Stressing the importance of practicing safe sex at each encounter perhaps will encourage the patient to refrain from having unprotected sex.

12. What responsibility do nurses have to HIV negative partners?

The knee jerk response to this question by some healthcare workers would be to notify the patients' partners that they have been exposed to HIV. However, partner notification has not been effective because of the long incubation period of HIV; the patient may have exposed numerous individuals through unprotected sex or needle sharing and it would be impossible to contact all partners involved. Also since illegal injection drug use is a felony in all 50 states, needle-sharing partners using illegal drugs would not want their activity identified by public officials for fear of prosecution.

Healthcare providers should encourage the patient to disclose to his/her partners his/her HIV status. Also referring the patient to peer educators or HIV organizations that address this issue may assist the patient to make an informed decision as to how to inform his/her current or future partners of his/her HIV status.

Tension exists between maintaining confidentiality and protecting individuals with HIV-AIDS. Both the American Medical Association and the American Psychological Association support the following roles for the physician and the psychologist:

1. attempt to persuade the infected patient to cease endangering the third party;

2. if persuasion fails, notify authorities; and

3. if the authorities take no action, notify the endangered third party (Fletcher, Lombardo, Marshall, & Miller, 1997).

13. Can a pregnant woman refuse HIV testing?

Yes, a pregnant woman can refuse HIV testing. Now you may question why any woman would refuse to know her HIV status in order to protect her unborn child. There are many implications that a woman may face if she discovers she is HIV positive. She and her child would have the stigma of having HIV. She may face rejection by her partner or family. Also she may be at risk for violent attacks.

This being said it is recommended that all pregnant women be tested for HIV as a routine part of prenatal care. The American College of Obstetrics and Gynecology and the American Academy of Pediatrics have supported routine universal prenatal HIV testing. However, if a routine HIV test is done in the prenatal period, the mother's rights to refuse the test will be violated. If routine HIV testing occurs, the mother may not even be aware that an HIV test was done, so her right to autonomy will be violated.

14. What is the nurse's responsibility if the HIV-infected mother refuses to be tested?

An HIV-infected pregnant woman who refuses HIV testing may perceive that being tested for HIV is a threat to her either physically or socially if the result is positive. The nurse's responsibility is to determine the reason the woman is refusing the test. If the woman is not willing to discuss her reasons, the nurse should educate the mother on how HIV can affect both herself and her newborn. The mother should be informed that babies who receive treatment for HIV during delivery and after birth and whose mothers receive medications in the prenatal period, have a 99% chance of not having HIV. On the other hand in the absence of HIV treatment during pregnancy, the risk of a baby acquiring the virus from an infected mother ranges from 15 to 25% in industrialized countries and 25 to 35% in developing countries.

15. What ethical issues arise in testing an HIV vaccine on HIV-positive patients?

At present the vaccine has proven ineffective. Nurses working with patients involved in HIV vaccine research must inform the patients of the risks of participating in such research. Vaccine trials pose unique risks to the participants. Participants may be prevented from participating in future vaccine trials, and vaccines developed later may be less effective for them.

In addition, because participants may react positively to certain HIV antibody tests, they may also face limits on international travel and ineligibility for certain governmental jobs (e.g., Peace Corps, Foreign Service, Job Corps, and the military) even if their seroconversion does not represent true infection. Participation in some trials may identify the subject as someone at high risk of contracting HIV, an identification that may entail numerous difficulties. Although researchers always have an obligation to protect the confidentiality of the information they collect, this duty is particularly important in HIV vaccine trials because of the high stakes if confidentiality is breached.

16. What responsibility do industrialized countries have to developing countries in supplying medication to treat HIV?

Developing countries such as sub-Saharan Africa are most affected by HIV/AIDS. It is estimated that 29.4 million people are living with HIV/AIDS and approximately 3.5 million new infections occurred in 2002. In the past year the epidemic has claimed the lives of an estimated 2.4 million Africans. The impact of HIV on sub-Saharan Africa has been devastating, affecting the labor force, households, and enterprises. HIV/AIDS has had a major effect on the African economy, and in turn this affects Africa's ability to cope with the epidemic.

Industrialized countries have the moral responsibility to provide funding to halt the devastating effect of HIV on developing nations. A Global Fund to fight AIDS, tuberculosis, and malaria indicated that $7–10 billion is required annually to tackle the HIV epidemic in developing nations. The Global Fund has awarded $1.5 billion to developing nations to provide health care, of which Africa is being given 62%. As of June 2003, only nine African countries had actually received money from the fund for HIV/AIDS, and the total distributed for Africa was only $5.8 million. Without the required money, testing and counseling programs will not be developed, condoms will not be distributed, and antiretroviral medications will not be available to the neediest citizens of the world.

17. Is it ethical to do HIV research on the populations of developing countries if those countries are unable to provide medications to HIV-infected people once the research is completed?

A major issue in international research is making therapies available to developing countries once they are shown to be effective. Researchers, research sponsors, and international organizations are trying to negotiate with drug manufacturers and host country governments to make therapies available at affordable prices. This may entail discounted prices, licensing agreements to manufacture the drug in a developing country, or other strategies.

However, the appropriateness of providing antiretroviral therapies in developing countries, particularly Africa, has been the subject of debate. Some have argued that the severity of the AIDS epidemic in the developing world requires that antiretroviral therapies be provided to those affected by it. Others have argued that the lack of healthcare infrastructure makes provision of these drugs inappropriate at this time.

To improve the healthcare infrastructure and facilitate drug distribution, Botswana, in conjunction with Bill & Melinda Gates Foundation and Merck & Company has developed a new initiative that would provide for a comprehensive delivery system of drugs and a prevention program for HIV/AIDS. The Botswana Comprehensive HIV/AIDS Partnership will try to advance prevention, healthcare access, patient management, and treatment of HIV in Botswana, where an estimated 29% of the adult population is HIV positive. Focusing on improving existing healthcare capabilities for people with HIV/AIDS, the project will start with awareness, education, and voluntary testing and counseling programs. As the project advances, access to HIV treatment and care will expand significantly, in step with healthcare infrastructure improvements, including treatments for tuberculosis, HIV-related opportunistic infections, and HIV infections.

Boehringer-Ingelheim said it will donate medication for the prevention of mother-to-child transmission, and Unilever PLC will contribute expertise in setting up distribution systems and communication and awareness campaigns. The success of the Botswana Comprehensive HIV/AIDS Partnership will serve as a model for other African countries.

18. Do you believe that harm reduction practices such as needle exchange and providing condoms in schools are ethical?

Teens are the fastest growing group at risk for HIV. Two teens are infected with HIV every hour in the United States. One in four new HIV cases in the United States occurs in people under the age of 22.

I believe not offering harm reduction practices is unethical. Whether the community or society wants to acknowledge it, high school kids are having unprotected sex and using drugs. The number of teens who have positive Gonorrhea and Chlamydia tests is astounding. Teens between the ages of 15 and 19 are four times as likely as 30–44-year-olds to develop one repeat infection and five times as likely to be reinfected with Chlamydia and Gonorrhea at least twice. Teens also are using injection drugs and sharing needles. Needle exchange programs have proven effective in reducing the spread of HIV.

I am not a proponent of teens having sex or using drugs, but by offering students condoms, providing them with STD counseling and a needle exchange program, nurses can empower teenagers to make informed decisions regarding sex and drug use.

19. Should an HIV-positive person be held accountable if he/she knowingly has unprotected sex?

Knowingly putting another at risk for HIV is reprehensible. However, criminal prosecution of HIV-infected individuals practicing unsafe sex is not the way to prevent transmission of HIV. Public officials should encourage at risk people to be tested for HIV with the assurance that their privacy will be respected. I believe that when people living with HIV believe that their rights of autonomy and self-determination will not be violated, they will be forthcoming about their HIV status to their sexual partners and condom use will increase.

20. There is much misinformation and mistrust among the African American population regarding the origin of HIV and the current availability of treatment. How can healthcare workers gain the trust of the African American community?

I have encountered an African American patient who has stated that he believes HIV was intentionally planted in the African American community by the government to eliminate their race. If I have had one patient who openly spoke about this to me, how many more African Americans actually believe this to be true? If a patient believes that the goal of the government is to annihilate his race, what are the chances he is going to adhere to a treatment regimen?

The U.S. Public Health Services study on "Untreated Syphilis in the Negro Male" (the infamous Tuskegee Study) is often cited as the prime example of why African Americans mistrust the medical community. However, other research suggests that this mistrust stems from a centuries-long history of medical mistreatment and abuse.

Nurses can help reduce the African American community's mistrust of medical treatment by providing culturally sensitive medical information. Also, refer patients to African American HIV organizations to provide support and counseling such as Blacks Educating Blacks About Sexual Health Issues (BEBASHI).

21. Can family members prevent healthcare workers from telling the patient his/her HIV status?

Withholding a person's HIV status at the request of the family is denying the patient his/her right of self-determination. In this instance, the nurse must act as a patient advocate. The nurse should inform the family that it is in the patient's best interest that the patient knows the diagnosis and prognosis, especially since with treatment the individual could live a long life. Knowing the truth about his/her clinical illness, the patient can make informed decisions in determining the course of treatment or refuse treatment.

RESOURCES

AIDS and the Law. (1998). Your rights in Pennsylvania (3rd ed.). Philadelphia: Aids Law Project of Pennsylvania. [Booklet].

AVERT.org. (2002). HIV and AIDS in Africa, Worldwide HIV and AIDS Statistics. http://www.avert.org

Daily reproductive health report: Public health & education. High reinfection rates of Chlamydia among teens highlight need for screening, counseling, study says. (2001, June 21). Retrieved from http://www.kaisernetwork.org

Ferriman, A. (2001). Doctors demand immediate access to antiretroviral drugs in Africa. *British Medical Journal, 322,* 1012.

Fletcher, J., Lombardo, P., Marshall, M., & Miller, F. (1997). *Introduction to clinical ethics.* Hagerstown, MD: University Publishing Group.

Global Health Council Webmaster. (2000, July 13). Global Health Council: General Health News. Africa: Botswana. Retrieved from http://www.reutershealth.com/archive/2000/07/eline/links/20000707elin026html

Gosten, L. (2000). National policy on HIV-infected healthcare workers questions. *Journal of the American Medical Association, 284*(15), 1965–1970.

Jurgens, R. Canadian HIV/AIDS Legal Network. Testing and confidentiality: Final report. Retrieved from http://www.AIDSLAW.CA/HIV

Kapos, S. (2003, April 20). HIV compromise wins support. *Chicago Tribune,* p. 1.

Kirton, C. (2003). *ANAC's core curriculum for HIV/AIDS nursing* (2nd ed.). London: Sage Publications.

Scherzer, M. (1998, October). The Body: An HIV and AIDS information resource-HIV and insurance: Some questions and answers. Retrieved from http://www.thebody.com/scherzer/nivens98.html

Wolf, L. E., & Lo, B. (2001). HIV InSite knowledge base. In ethical dimensions of HIV/AIDS. S. Burrowes (Ed.). University of California, San Francisco. Retrieved from http://www.hivinsite.ucsf.edu/insite.jsp?page=kbr-08-01-07&doc=kb=08-01-05#

Chapter 12

Diseases Where Patient Behaviors Are a Key Factor: Ethical Issues

Doris V. Chaplin

1. **Should healthcare dollars be spent on individuals diagnosed with lung cancer who continue to smoke and chew tobacco?**

Millions of dollars have been spent educating the public about the causal relationship between cigarette smoking and cancer. Today, 24% of the U.S. population continues to smoke. Nicotine addiction is a difficult drug dependency to break. If we stopped treating this individual, then in order to be fair, we would also have to stop treating other individuals with addictions. However, addiction is a disease, and as other diseases, needs to be treated.

2. *Case:* **A patient is diagnosed with terminal lung cancer. Can I deny him cigarettes and encourage his family to make them unavailable to him?**

The third statement in "The Patient's Bill of Rights" states that the patient has "the right to make decisions about his care." It is the nurse's duty to inform the patient of the additional negative consequences of his actions, but ultimately he remains the guardian of his personal decisions. Perhaps this could be a time to offer him other choices, such as the nicotine patch, to help him cope with withdrawal.

3. Should individuals continue to receive pain medication to control their angina when they refuse to stop smoking?

Can we prove that cigarette smoking is the only cause of the angina pain? Do we know if other equal stressors are depriving the patient of the oxygen needed? Denying the patient pain medication is unethical, as well as cruel. The most we can do is to help the individual face the fact that continuing to smoke will only increase the severity of the problem and provide information on how to stop smoking.

4. Should an individual with HIV who acquired the disease by homosexual practices be given the same level of treatment as an individual who acquired HIV unknowingly through an adulterous homosexual spouse?

Respect for a person is the most fundamental human right. It requires that each person be respected as a unique individual equal to another person. As a caregiver, you may be angry at the spouse's unfaithfulness and lies that led to the patient's getting HIV from an adulterous spouse, yet you cannot treat this patient any differently than the one who acquired HIV because of a homosexual preference. If you find yourself contemplating discriminating the quality of care provided in either situation, it would be appropriate to examine your biases and perhaps discuss your feelings with a trusted colleague. According to the *Code*, "Nurses must examine the conflicts arising between their personal and professional values" (p. 19).

5. Should individuals who are habitually non-compliant with their prescribed medicine pay a higher premium on their health insurance?

Possibly paying higher premiums for health insurance could motivate an individual to adhere to treatment regimens. However, it has never been proven that having this knowledge changes the behavior of an individual. Much research has been done on patient's non-compliance with medications; two studies are reported here. First, beliefs about medications were related to adherence: individuals who believed that the drug was necessary had higher adherence and individuals with more concerns over the drug's long-term effects or side effects demonstrated low adherence. Patients engage in an implicit cost-benefit analysis. Therefore, the nurse needs to engage in this dialogue with the patient to foster compliance (Home & Weinman, 1999). Second, adherence to medication regimen was related to establishing a medication-taking pattern—the same time and place each day (Johnson, Williams, & Marshall, 1999).

6. **A patient sustained a neurological injury because he refused to wear his helmet while riding his motorcycle. Should healthcare dollars be spent on an individual who refuses to wear safety devices?**

Yes, in spite of the unwise behavior, we are to provide care "irrespective of the nature of the health problem." Laws are established to protect people from harming self or others. As healthcare providers, we are obligated to continue providing care while reinforcing to the patient, family, and friends the long-term burden these injuries place on society.

7. **Should there be a health patrol policing negative health practices of individuals with repeated abusive behaviors and then deny them health benefits?**

A democratic society prohibits this type of policing. This type of policing would open a gate for abuse. Patients are unable to change self-abusive behaviors for a number of reasons; the nurse's role is to support patients in stopping these behaviors. Addiction, depression, and other psychological disorders as well as poverty are just a few reasons that make these behaviors difficult to overcome. Far better than policing is a nurse providing compassion, education, and support.

8. *Case:* **The parents of an obese 8-year-old patient do not support their child in losing weight; in fact, they keep a significant amount of high-fat and high-sugar foods around the house. Should they be penalized by paying higher health insurance?**

We cannot penalize the parents by having them pay more for their healthcare coverage. First, we must help the family see the repercussions of their child's eating behavior, then engage the parents and child in nutrition and possibly family counseling. Since the evidence for the adverse effects on health is overwhelming and indisputable, help them see the health consequences the obesity is having, including any psychological problems. Do not focus on the high-sugar and high-fat food, but discuss other ways they can support the child.

9. Should there be a three-strike law that cancels an individual's health insurance because he/she refuses to change his/her habitually abusive behavior?

Society is obligated to take care of people who are ill. It is a belief in this society that we are obligated to do what is right to help a person, in spite of the person's repeated abusive behavior. This practice is evident by the many rehabilitation and prevention programs, as well as halfway houses that exist in this country. According to the ANA (2001) *Code*, nurses have a responsibility "to assist in efforts to educate the public . . . facilitate healthy lifestyles, and participate in institutional and legislative efforts to promote health and meet national health objectives" (p. 24). Nurses also have a responsibility to remove barriers to health such as poverty, violence, and unsafe living conditions that play a part in individuals' choosing abusive behaviors.

10. Why are we paying for bypass surgery when heart-healthy programs can prevent heart disease?

It is true heart-healthy programs affect a normal cholesterol, blood sugar, and blood pressure levels, but individuals must be motivated to enter such programs. Even with individuals who have had a heart attack, only 29% complete cardiac rehab. Clinicians have researched for years trying to find the key to getting people to change destructive lifestyles, but today people still choose bypass surgery over changing lifestyle.

Motivational interviewing is a client-centered counseling approach for eliciting behavior change by helping clients explore and resolve their ambivalence. The approach helps the client make the argument for change by tapping into the client's intrinsic motivation and core values. Perhaps nurses using this approach could help patients choose a healthier lifestyle.

11. Should individuals in prison because of murder, without chance of parole, become candidates for organ donation or have the opportunity to be organ recipients?

A criminal gives up his political rights and citizenship privileges. However, he maintains his personal rights; therefore, as a criminal he can make the decision as to whether to donate his organs. The law states that the criminal has a right to receive any medical treatment that is deemed medically necessary. Almost 30 years ago, the Supreme Court ruled that prisoners were entitled to receive adequate health care. Transplantation is treated as part of basic medical services in this country. Any policy that would award lower priority to prisoners would be based on some sense that prisoners are less valuable members of society and would introduce the notion of social worth to the entire transplant system. Should other members of society who act irresponsibly and make self-destructive lifestyle choices be excluded too?

Crimes deemed sufficiently heinous warrant the death penalty, otherwise imprisonment is the way criminals pay their debt. Some ethicists argue that certain crimes, such as first-degree murder and repeat sexual offenders (whether rapist or pedophile), should be candidates for exclusion. Obviously, these behaviors are not in the same league as binge drinking, smoking, or obesity.

12.   Should food producers be held accountable for producing food that is rich with substances that research demonstrates negatively contributes to health (e.g., estrogen-rich food causing cancer)?

Labels that clearly alert consumers to the ingredients would put the choice in their hands. Now, genetically altered food is only labeled when it is shipped outside the U.S. Holding the tobacco companies accountable for the illness caused by cigarette smoking sets a precedent for holding these manufacturers accountable. Initially, the cigarette companies had to label the cigarette pack to indicate disease-causing properties. Should we not at least require this of food enriched with cancer-causing substances?

13.   Should foods rich in additives that increase the risk of cancer and other major diseases be banned from the grocery stores?

People in the United States suffer many illnesses because of the food that they eat, as well as the amount of food that they eat. However, we are a country that believes strongly in choice, but at least let us educate Americans on harmful additives and on how to eat more natural foods.

14.   Should known addicts be refused health care unless they enroll in a program that modifies their risky behaviors?

Most people do not know that the rate of relapse for individuals with addiction is similar to other rates of relapse with chronic diseases like diabetes or chronic obstructive pulmonary disease (COPD). As the ANA *Code* says, "the nursing profession is committed to promoting the health, welfare and safety of all people" (p. 23). The nurse's obligation is to help individuals suffering from addiction to obtain the best treatment possible, just as he/she would for any other illness.

15. **Case: A patient has a long history of back pain. He has refused to wear a back brace at work or learn the stretching and strengthening exercises the physical therapist taught him. Why can we not refuse to treat such patients?**

    Every patient is entitled to care regardless of race, creed, or harmful behavior. The cycle is vicious, but we must keep prodding and teaching what is correct as the ANA (2001) *Code* always governs nursing practice.

16. **Case: A patient has had uncontrolled diabetes for over a year. Should she not automatically be a candidate for an insulin pump to assist her to better control her HgA$_{LC}$ resulting in fewer disease complications?**

    The patient certainly is a candidate for an insulin pump and with a physician's order and appropriate training, she could be ready to use the pump. Studies do support the idea that there are less long-term complications with individuals using a pump because they can achieve good control over their blood sugar. Most people would never go back to daily injections once they have used the pump. It is as small as a pager and delivers units of insulin continuously through a small tube. Since you only change the site and infusion set every three days and the process takes only 15 minutes, there is a high level of acceptance.

17. **A patient with End Stage Renal Disease (ESRD) refuses to make dietary and lifestyle changes. Should he be denied access to health care?**

Individuals with ESRD generally have strict dietary guidelines. In research (Oka et al., 1999), we found that support from family members and nurses was significantly related to dietary compliance. Nurses working with dialysis patients should remember to use their influence to support patients. Support groups are often available for patients with this diagnosis and can provide further support and ideas from patients who have lived with the disease for many years.

RESOURCES

Adams, M. (2004, July 19). Is obesity a choice or a disease? *News Target*. www.news target.com/001416.html

Bodenheimer, T., Lorig, K., Holman, H., & Grumbach, K. (2002). Patient self-management of chronic diseases in primary care. *Journal of the American Medical Association, 288*(19), 2469–2475.

Greenlund, K. J., Giles, W. H., Keenan, N. L., Croft, J. B., & Mensah, G. A. (2002). Physician advice, patient actions, and health-related quality of life in secondary prevention of stroke through diet and exercise. *Stroke, 33*(2), 565–570.

Horne, R., & Weinman, J. (1999). Patients' beliefs about prescribed medicines and their role in adherence to treatment in chronic physical illness. *Journal of Psychosomatic Research, 47*(6), 555–567.

Johnson, M. J., Williams, M., & Marshall, E. (1999). Adherent and nonadherent medication-taking in elderly hypertensive patients. *Clinical Nursing Research, 8*(4), 318–335.

Koffman, D. M., Bazzarre, T., Mosca, L., Redberg, R., Schmid, T., & Wattigney, W. A. (2001). An evaluation of Choose to Move 1999: An American Heart Association physical activity program for women. *Archives of Internal Medicine, 161*(18), 2193–2199, 2271–2272.

Oka, M., Chaboyer, W., & Molzahn, A. (1999). Dietary behaviors and sources of support in hemodialysis patients. *Clinical Nursing Research, 8*(4), 302–310.

Thorpe, M. (2003). Motivational interviewing and dietary behavior change. *Journal of the American Dietetic Association, 103*(2), 150–151.

Chapter 13

Long-Term Care Patients: Ethical Issues

Diane Stillman

1. How do we decide if residents can make their own health-care decisions?

In the area of healthcare decisions, it is imperative to respect personal autonomy.

Unless there is significant evidence to the contrary, it is assumed that a person, including a resident of a nursing home, is able to make his/her own healthcare decisions. There are two terms used when describing an individual's ability to make decisions: competence and decision-making capacity. Competence is the legal ability to make one's own decisions and is determined by a legal hearing in which evidence is presented that the person is able to manage his/her financial or personal affairs without risk to his/her safety. While there are situations that require a legal determination of competence (such as a person who is not able to care for him/herself refusing placement in a nursing home), in most cases this legal determination is not necessary as the individual is cooperative with the decisions of the family.

Decision-making capacity refers to an individual's ability to make a specific decision and is a healthcare judgment, not a legal one. Decision-making capacity is situation specific and may vary over time. Thus, a resident may be able to decide who he/she wants involved in his/her care but may not be able to decide whether he/she wishes to have surgery or he/she may be lucid enough to make a reasoned decision at one point in the day and not at another time.

In order to make an informed decision individuals must

- know they have a choice,

- understand the medical situation, recommended treatment, risks and benefits, and likely consequences, and

- maintain a reasonable amount of decision-making stability over time.

Decision-making capacity is usually determined by the resident's primary care provider. However, if the nursing staff believes that a resident who is able to participate in healthcare decisions is being excluded, it is their responsibility to advocate for the resident's autonomy.

2. What is the difference between a responsible party, a guardian, and a power of attorney?

Determining who is responsible for making decisions for a nursing home resident who lacks decision-making capacity can be confusing. There are different designations used in long-term care that denote different legal and personal relationships.

a. Responsible Party: A person who usually signs the 140 Section 3: Ethical Issues With Disenfranchised Patients admissions papers with the resident and is the contact for financial concerns and care planning issues. If a resident is not able to make decisions it is often assumed by the facility that this person is responsible for decision making. Legally, the next-of-kin would be the person called on for healthcare decisions if a resident lacks decision-making capacity and has no living will, power of attorney, or guardian. If the responsible party is not next-of-kin, the facility must document why the next of kin is not making these decisions.

b. Guardian: A person appointed by a court of law to assume responsibility for the financial and/or personal decisions of another adult who is deemed incompetent.

c. Power of Attorney: Person named by the resident when the resident still has decision-making capacity to handle the resident's financial and/or healthcare decisions should the individual become incapacitated. In order for a power of attorney to be able to make healthcare decisions for an incapacitated person he/she must be a Durable Power of Attorney for Health Care.

d. Health Care Proxy: Many Living Wills require the signer to name a person to make healthcare decisions if he/she is unable to do so. This person is called the Health Care Proxy.

It is important to remember that a guardian, durable power of attorney, and health care proxy all have legal standing as the persons appointed either by the courts or by the resident to make decisions. The decisions of these individuals would supersede that of the responsible party or even the next-of-kin.

3. What do you do if a resident and his/her family disagree on care decisions?

In most cases, nursing home residents involve their family in care decisions even if they are capable of making these decisions independently. As most residents of nursing homes are in frail health, the support of family is important to residents when making difficult decisions. However, there are times when family members disagree with the choices of their loved one and they usually bring their concerns to the nursing home staff.

The staff must support the autonomy of the resident, even if a family member has been very involved in the life of a resident. It should be clear to all concerned that the patient's choices will be respected and communicated to all members of the healthcare team. There may be times when a resident no longer wants health information shared with his/her family and this wish for privacy must be respected by staff.

When a resident lacks decision-making capacity, disagreements between the resident and his/her family regarding care can be more serious. This is especially true when a resident is making decisions that may cause serious harm to him/herself. When a resident has not been deemed incompetent by a court of law, a family member, even one with durable power of attorney, cannot override the wishes of the resident. Most of the time family members avoid legal confrontation by working with staff to convince the incapacitated person to accept help in making safe decisions regarding his/her care. However, if the person cannot be convinced and is unable to act in his/her own best interest, the family may seek a legal hearing to establish competence and appoint a guardian. In emergencies, this can be done very quickly.

4. To what extent should someone with dementia be involved in decisions affecting his/her own care?

The simple answer to this is that every person should be encouraged to participate in decisions regarding his/her own care. The Nursing Home Reform Act of 1987 upholds this principle by emphasizing that residents have the right to self-determination, including the right to participate in care planning and the right to refuse treatment. While residents with dementia may not be able to understand all care decisions, recent research has shown that even residents with moderate to severe dementia can often express consistent preferences in care and consistently name a person whom he/she would wish to make decisions for him/her. If a resident is able to make his/her wishes and preferences known, these should be respected whenever possible.

5. What can be done if a resident or his/her family decides on a course of action that staff at the facility do not think is in the resident's best interests?

In cases where the resident still has decision-making capacity, the staff must respect the resident's autonomy. While this may be difficult for the staff, it is important to recognize the importance of individual self-determination and continue to provide the resident with excellent care and support.

In cases where the resident lacks decision-making capacity, the facility must decide whether it is necessary to intervene on the resident's behalf. Often a useful first step is to arrange a meeting with nursing staff, social services, and the resident's physician to discuss the problem and consider possible courses of action. If this fails to resolve the problem, the issue can be brought to the facility's ethics committee. Last, if the problem persists and the staff believes it is necessary to intervene to prevent harm to the resident, legal proceedings can be instituted to challenge the decisions made by the family. While the nature of the legal issues differs depending on the legal status of the decision maker (guardian versus responsible party versus power of attorney), the basic steps toward resolution are the same.

6. What role, if any, should the staff of a long-term care facility have in assisting a resident with completion of a living will?

The Patients Self Determination Act (PSDA) of 1990 requires all healthcare agencies that receive federal funding to recognize advance directives. Facilities are responsible for educating residents on their right to institute advance directives, supplying appropriate forms to record advance directives, and making this information available in the healthcare record. Unfortunately, there is often confusion as to whom, if anyone, should assist the resident in completing the advance directive. The concern over appearing coercive has often led to an extreme reluctance to explain the document and its terms.

While it is appropriate for a facility to avoid pressuring residents to complete advance directives, it is widely recommended by those involved in end-of-life care that individuals be guided through the process of advance care planning. Ideally, there should be members of the staff, usually social workers, trained to assist families in this regard. These staff should explain the process, review the terms used in the advance directive, and discuss the fact that the advance directives can be changed at any time. Ideally, the resident should also be encouraged to discuss his/her values, fears, and wishes for end-of-life care. Residents should be encouraged to talk with their family, clergy person, and healthcare providers about the decisions outlined in the advance directive. Ideally, an advance directive should be completed in a series of conversations rather than being rushed through in one sitting and should be reviewed periodically to ensure it still represents the wishes of the resident. Samples of advance directive forms can be found at www.uslivingwillregistry.com.

7. At some facilities, families complete a living will for the resident. Is this legally binding?

The practice of having a person who is responsible for making decisions for an incapacitated person (such as a healthcare proxy or next-of-kin) complete a living will is becoming more common in nursing homes. While this practice could be a helpful way to document treatment preferences before a crisis arises, it is not a legally binding document. A Living Will is by definition completed by the resident before he/she loses decision-making capacity and, thus, represents the expressed wishes of the resident. The document completed by families is not a Living Will but a tool to document understanding of the wishes of the resident regarding advance care planning.

8. Why are long-term care facilities now striving to be "restraint free"?

Restraints are estimated to be used on as many as 500,000 frail, aged, and disabled persons in the United States. A restraint is any device used to restrict the freedom of a person including side rails, belts, vests, hand mitts, and Geri chairs. These devices protect frail or confused residents from falls and other accidents. However, research has demonstrated that rather than protect residents from harm, restraints increase the likelihood of serious injury. In fact, as many as 200 people die each year because they strangle or suffocate in restraints even if the devices are applied correctly. Restraints have also been shown to contribute to avoidable decline in ability to walk, decreased muscle tone, contracture formation, and increased incidence of pressure sores, infections, delirium, agitation, depression, constipation, and incontinence.

The Nursing Home Reform Act of 1987 states the resident has the right to be free from physical or chemical restraints imposed for purposes of discipline or convenience and not required to treat the resident's medical symptoms. Before restraining a resident, the facility must demonstrate the presence of a specific medical symptom that would require the use of restraints and how the use of the restraint would (1) treat the cause of the symptom and, (2) assist the resident in reaching the highest level of physical and psychosocial well-being. When restraints are evaluated with these criteria in mind, it is clear there is little or no justification for restraint use among most of the nursing home population.

9. When is the use of psychoactive medications considered "chemical restraint"?

A medication is considered a chemical restraint if it is administered for the primary or explicit purpose of reducing an individual's functional capacity (sedation). This is forbidden by law if used for discipline or convenience. The drugs usually targeted as potential chemical restraints are antipsychotic medications (e.g., Zyprexa, Risperdal, Haldol) and anxiolytics (e.g., Xanax, Ativan). While these drugs can be very helpful in controlling symptoms of neurological and psychiatric illnesses, such as hallucinations or anxiety, they may not be used to control irritating behavior or for convenience of the staff. Thus, it is important both ethically and legally to ensure that these medications are being used for specified symptoms and that the reason for use and any adverse effects are well documented.

10. What are ways that staff can demonstrate a respect for the Residents' Bill of Rights?

Most states require that nursing homes display a Patients' Bill of Rights. This Bill of Rights varies by state but in general includes:

a. The right to be fully informed

b. The right to make independent decisions

c. The right to privacy and confidentiality

d. The right to dignity, respect, and freedom

e. The right to security of possessions

f. The right to be transferred or discharged

g. The right to complain

h. The right to visits

These rights should be affirmed by staff members and recognized as the minimum standard at which ethical care should be judged. These tenets emphasize that a person continues to have the right to be treated with dignity and respect and afforded with all possible freedom despite the disability that requires him/her to reside in a nursing home. Affirming these rights includes such everyday acts as ensuring privacy before providing personal care, honoring refusal of treatments, and speaking in a respectful, adult tone. These simple acts convey to the residents that they are valued individuals in the community and allow them to maintain a sense of dignity and control in difficult circumstances.

11. How should staff handle residents' expressions of sexuality?

Sexuality is a fundamental human need common to all people. There is no evidence that this need disappears with increased age and disability, but the obstacles to sexual expression in the nursing home setting are numerous. The most formidable barriers to sexual expression are discomfort of the staff with the topic of sexuality in older adults and the lack of privacy. Married residents must, by law, be provided with a shared room if desired. Residents who are not married and express a desire for privacy should be provided with a private place to be alone that is appropriate for sexual expression. Additionally, a person who is qualified to educate them about engaging in sexual behavior in a safe way given their physical limitations should counsel residents.

12. What is the role of an ombudsman and his/her relationship to ethical issues in long-term care?

Ombudsman is a Swedish word that means "One who speaks on behalf of another." Every state is required to have an Ombudsman Program that addresses complaints and advocates for improvements in the long-term care system. There are approximately 1,000 paid ombudsmen and 8,000 certified volunteers nationwide.

Ombudsman programs receive individual complaints by or on behalf of residents of nursing homes and assisted living facilities and work to resolve these complaints. The phone number for the local Ombudsman program is required to be clearly posted in nursing homes for the information of residents and family members. Unfortunately, many long-term care facilities view the Ombudsman as an adversary. This happens because the Ombudsman is called in to investigate complaints of abuse or substandard care. However, it is not only the resident or family who may request assistance from the Ombudsman in resolving difficult issues. The administration of long-term care institutions may also contact the Ombudsman when there is a particularly difficult issue to be resolved.

When ethical issues arise, the primary role of the Ombudsman is to advocate for the resident. Ombudsmen are trained in conflict resolution and their focus is ensuring that residents' rights and wishes are respected. When the resident is cognitively impaired, an Ombudsman can also facilitate discussions with family members or significant others to ascertain what the resident would want if he/she were able to participate in decision making. This is especially helpful when making difficult end-of-life decisions in which the family is conflicted.

13. How might a Residents' Council address an ethical concern?

A residents' council is an independent, organized group of persons living in a nursing home who meet on a regular basis to discuss concerns, develop suggestions, and plan activities. Federal laws give residents the right to meet as a council and mandate that they have the right to meet privately. Typically, councils meet at least monthly and have an elected board of officers. They meet with the administration of the facility or, if desired by council, they can meet with staff.

Laws, rules, and policies set by the government and the nursing home administration heavily control the lives of nursing home residents. Residents' councils allow residents to maintain an active role in the decisions that affect them. There are many benefits to an active residents' council including improved communication, better identification of problems within the home, increased participation in developing activities within the facility, and development of friendships between residents.

Residents' councils are also called upon to address an ethical concern that is affecting the population. For example, if staff members discuss confidential resident information in open areas, a resident could bring this concern to the council for discussion and recommendations. During the meeting, the residents could discuss the need for privacy and dignity and perhaps even formulate a more acceptable alternative such as staff using the conference room when it is necessary to discuss confidential information. The council officials could then bring their concerns and proposed alternative to administration.

14. What is the right thing to do when residents' wishes conflict with Federal regulations: for example, the resident likes to sit on the floor to watch TV?

The Federal regulations establish that the resident has a right to a dignified existence, self-determination, and communication with and access to persons and services inside and outside the nursing home. However, in an effort to protect residents, there are some specific provisions emphasized by state inspectors that may conflict with residents' wishes. For example, there are residents who enjoy sitting in the hallway rather than in a room, who wish you to enter their room without knocking, or who want to sit or lay on the floor.

Since the facility is the resident's home, resident wishes should be respected unless there is a compelling reason for the facility to intervene (i.e., unless a resident is in danger of harming themselves or others). In order to satisfy regulators the facility team must explore the reasons that the resident wishes to engage in the activity and ascertain whether there may be a preferable alternative. Lastly, the Ombudsman may be very helpful in determining how to best meet the resident's needs and still adhere to all necessary federal regulations.

Thus, if a resident wishes to sit on the floor, staff should discuss this choice with the resident to determine whether this is truly a preferred pattern or whether the resident has a need that is not being met. The facility should discuss any potential risks of the activity such as the floors not being as clean as a chair or the possibility the resident could fall when getting up from the floor. Then, the facility should work with the resident to outline an area where he/she may sit on the floor without being a hazard to other residents such as against the wall in his/her room. Last, all these discussions should be documented in the healthcare record and the resident's preferences should be noted on the care plan. If a patient wishes to have his/her family involved, or is unable to make independent decisions, family members should be invited to participate in this process. If the facility is at all concerned regarding whether the devised plan would be acceptable to state regulators, it is wise to call the Department of Health or the Ombudsman for guidance.

15. Should the staff handle the needs of a resident under 65 differently than those of residents who are over 65?

While the average age of nursing home residents is approximately 84 years and over 90% of nursing home residents are over 65, some nursing home residents are younger. There are many debilitating diseases and conditions including multiple sclerosis, cerebral palsy, acquired immune deficiency syndrome (AIDS), psychiatric illness, and cancer, which can require even young adults to reside in long-term care facilities providing skilled nursing care. Therefore, it is necessary that staff be knowledgeable about healthcare needs and developmental stages across the life span.

However, while it is important to be sensitive to the fact that age may affect a resident's needs and concerns, it is also important not to make assumptions about a resident's needs based solely on age. While issues of lost livelihood, body image, separation from children, and need for intimacy are often identified as concerns of younger residents, many older residents also continue to have these concerns as well. When planning care it is always best to involve the resident and family in identifying needs and concerns and then individualize the plan of care based on these needs and concerns.

16. What should be done if a resident expresses a desire to eat regular food even though he/she has a swallowing difficulty and is at risk for aspiration?

The nursing home must respect the resident's right of self-determination. When a resident with a swallowing disorder wishes to forgo the diet recommended by speech therapy, it is necessary to ensure the resident is aware of the risks involved. This should involve documented communication between the resident, his/her physician, and speech therapist. However, once apprised of the risks, residents have the right to refuse the recommended diet and choose a regular diet.

The skilled nursing facility continues to have the responsibility to keep the resident as safe as possible. Therefore, it would be important to ask speech therapy to advise the resident of any techniques that would make the regular diet safer. Additionally, it should be recommended that the resident take meals in a dining room, supervised by nursing staff in case of choking. However, if the resident chooses to forgo these recommendations, his/her wishes should be respected.

The situation is, of course, more complicated if a resident is unable to make informed decisions about his/her care. In this case, the surrogate decision maker should be notified of the request. The interdisciplinary care team should meet with the surrogate and any other family members who are involved and discuss the risks and benefits of allowing the resident to eat a regular diet. The family may decide to honor the patient's wishes and liberalize the diet. These conversations and any plans that are formulated must be well documented in the healthcare record.

17. Pain is often undertreated in the long-term care resident population. What are the ethical responsibilities of the nurse in managing a resident's pain?

The ethical principle of beneficence applies to a nurse's responsibility to ensure adequate management of distressing symptoms. The American Nurses Association (ANA) and the International Council of Nurses both include alleviation of suffering among their guiding ethical principles. The ANA (2001) *Code* states, "The nurse should provide interventions to relieve pain and other symptoms . . . " (p. 8).

Unfortunately, despite this clear ethical imperative, pain is common among nursing home residents and is often not assessed and is undertreated. There have been many studies in recent years that have described this problem. In one such study, Teno and colleagues (2001) reported that over 40% of residents in pain at an initial assessment were in severe pain 60 to 180 days later. Another study found that 26% of residents without cancer reported daily pain and that a quarter of these residents went untreated. Very old residents, members of minority populations, and those with severe cognitive impairment are at greatest risk for underevaluation and management of pain.

The most important aspect of effective pain control is adequate assessment. There are many assessment tools available for both cognitively intact and cognitively impaired residents.

Additionally, nurses and physicians may be concerned about using doses of opioid analgesics sufficient to control pain. This reluctance is often rooted in fears of promoting addiction, suppressing the respiratory response, or arousing the suspicions of state regulators. Proper education is necessary to ensure clinical staff members are aware that the risk of these events is extremely small when pain medications are used appropriately to treat pain.

18. How should the staff handle refusal of treatment whether it is refusal of medications or even refusal of personal care?

Residents have the right to refuse any treatment including hospitalization, medical testing, medications, and assistance with personal care. However, it is necessary to ensure that the resident has all the information needed to make a reasoned decision on these matters. When a resident is refusing treatment or care, it is necessary to inform the patient's primary care provider (PCP) that the resident is refusing the ordered treatment. Then the staff and the PCP must be sure to describe to the resident the possible risks of refusing treatment and document these discussions in the healthcare record. For a resident who is refusing hygiene, this becomes more complicated because this decision will affect others in the home and will be seen as negligence by state regulators. If discussions with the resident about the necessity of adequate hygiene do not result in an adequate solution, it may be necessary for the nursing home administration to consult with the Ombudsman and request assistance with resolution of the issue.

Refusal of care becomes more complicated when a resident is not competent to make informed decisions about his/her plan of care. In this case, the refusal needs to be discussed with the proxy decision maker who has the responsibility of weighing the benefits and burdens of treatment plans and making a decision on behalf of the resident. Often, there is no reasonable way to continue certain treatments with a cognitively impaired resident against his/her will.

When a resident who has a cognitive impairment refuses personal care, the team must look at the personal care approach being used and the time the resident refuses. Oftentimes, routines associated with personal hygiene can be frightening and disorienting for residents with dementia. There may be alterations in setting or staff approach that would increase cooperation with care. Once a successful routine has been established, it is important to document the preferred routine and follow that routine closely to best ensure cooperation in confused residents.

19. What can staff do to prevent resident-to-resident abuse or resident-to-staff abuse?

Nursing homes are ethically and legally responsible for protecting residents from abusive behavior by other residents. This includes resolving roommate problems in a prompt manner, properly addressing any problem behaviors that could lead to abuse, ensuring adequate supervision of residents known to exhibit aggressive or inappropriate behavior, and reporting all instances of resident-to-resident abuse to the state regulatory agency. Unfortunately, resident-to-resident abuse is thought to be widely underreported, as not all nursing home staff recognize that all suspicion of abuse (whether committed by staff, visitors, or other residents) must be reported in a prompt manner.

Nursing home staff, especially nursing assistants, frequently suffer abuse from impaired or angry residents because of their close daily contact. Many residents of nursing homes have dementia or psychiatric illnesses and others are angry and resentful because of their inability to live independently. It is common for nursing assistants to be yelled at, sworn at, mocked, hit, kicked, scratched, or touched in a sexual manner by residents. Derogatory racial remarks are also an all too common occurrence within nursing homes. It is imperative that all residents and families be made aware from the time of admission that such treatment of staff is unacceptable and will not be tolerated.

In 1996, OSHA published violence prevention guidelines for healthcare facilities. These guidelines are not mandatory but support OSHA's mandate that employees are entitled to a safe and healthy workplace. Nursing home administrators are encouraged to develop an action plan to minimize incidences of violence and plan interventions for when incidents do occur. Additionally, since some residents are unable to control their own behavior because of neurological or psychiatric illness, training programs for nursing assistants should be implemented which assist nursing assistants in developing appropriate strategies for preventing violent and aggressive reactions and handling incidences of abuse. Violence against caregivers in nursing homes, while not completely preventable given the high numbers of cognitively impaired residents, should not be considered an expected, tolerated, or accepted part of the job.

20.   What are staff responsibilities for reporting the abuse committed by other staff?

The Center for Medicare and Medicaid Services (CMS) defines abuse as "the willful infliction of injury, unreasonable confinement, intimidation, or punishment with resulting physical harm, pain, or mental anguish" (Requirements for States and Long Term Care Facilities, 1992). Resident abuse is both unethical and clearly illegal. Federal regulations require that long-term care facilities report all "alleged violations of abuse neglect, mistreatment, misappropriation of resident property, and injuries of unknown source"

(Requirements for States and Long Term Care Facilities, 1992) immediately to the appropriate state agency. Additionally, the CMS requires that the facility conduct an internal investigation of the alleged abuse and file a report with the state agency within 5 working days. There is some variability in state law as to whether nursing homes are required to contact law enforcement authorities with suspicion of abuse. It is important to note, however, that reporting of suspected crimes to law enforcement should be done immediately, and crimes committed in a nursing home should be no exception.

Despite the Federal requirements for reporting suspected abuse, a recent General Accounting Office report shows that many nursing homes fail to report promptly alleged physical and sexual abuse of residents, and few cases of abuse are prosecuted. Additionally the report found that local law enforcement reported rarely being called to a nursing home with reports of physical or sexual abuse. Additionally, few incidences of abuse were prosecuted in court as regulatory agencies varied in their policies for reporting findings of abuse to law enforcement agencies. As such, law enforcement often never is notified of abuse or is notified only after long delays, which hamper gathering of evidence for criminal proceedings.

While the legal obligations for reporting abuse have been outlined, it is important to note the ethical imperative to report abuse. Nurses are ethically responsible to protect residents from harm caused by staff, other residents, or visitors. In addition to exerting every effort to prevent abuse from occurring, all incidences of suspected abuse must be promptly reported to the facility administrator. Additionally, it is important to cooperate fully with all internal investigations of abuse as well as any review by state agencies or law enforcement.

21. What do families need to know in order to discuss or report ethical concerns regarding their loved ones?

As discussed earlier, state and Federal regulations outline residents' rights, which include rights to privacy, dignity, freedom from restraint, and freedom from association. Upon admission, all residents and their families should receive notification in writing of patients' rights, rules of the facility, and rules and regulations pertaining to patient conduct and responsibilities. This exchange provides a common ground for raising ethical questions and concerns with care.

Family members also need to be able to access those responsible for the resident's care such as the primary care provider, the charge nurse, the nurse manager, the dietitian, the rehabilitation personnel, social services, administration, and any outside providers who may play a significant role in care (e.g., hospice, clergy). Families should be encouraged to communicate openly and frequently with those staff members involved in residents' care. If the issues are not resolved, then they need to feel comfortable bringing concerns about the direct care providers to the appropriate manager or administrator. When difficult situations arise, it is important for families to know that they can meet with the care team as a whole to resolve issues and ensure proper ethical treatment of the resident.

When residents lack decision-making capacity, families should be encouraged to frame all ethical concerns by considering what the patient's wishes were when he/she was capable of expressing them. Even when an individual is unable to make an informed decision, every attempt should be made to respect the resident's autonomy by respecting any preferences for care that a person expressed before he/she was incapacitated. At times, the advice of the Ombudsman or even legal counsel may be necessary when there are particularly difficult and complex issues.

Residents with dementia or mental illness may lack the decision-making capacity to agree to a sexual relationship. In this case it is important that the staff ensure that no other person take advantage of the resident. Additionally, individuals with dementia or mental illness may act in a sexual way toward caregivers or other residents or masturbate in inappropriate locations. Residents who act in a sexually inappropriate way toward staff or other residents should be clearly told that it is not acceptable and redirected to a more appropriate behavior. When residents are found masturbating in public areas they should be brought to a private place where they may engage in this activity. Inappropriate behavior should be identified in the care plan and interventions to reduce this behavior should be introduced.

RESOURCES

Advance Directive Forms: http://www.uslivingwillresgistry.com/forms.shtm/

Bernabei, R., Gambesi, G., Lapane, K., Landi, F., Gatsonis, C., Dunlop, R., Lipsitz, L., Steel, K., & Mor, V. (1998). Management of pain in elderly patients with cancer. SAGE study group. (Systematic Assessment of Geriatric Drug Use via Epidemiology). *Journal of the American Medical Association, 279,* 1877–1882.

Mattiason, A., & Hemberg, M. (1998). Intimacy—Meeting needs and respecting privacy in the care of elderly people: What is a good moral attitude on the part of the nurse/caregiver? *Nursing Ethics, 5*(6), 527–534.

Nursing homes: More can be done to protect residents from abuse—GAO-02-312. http://www.gao.gov

OSHA guidelines for preventing workplace violence for health-care and social service workers. OSHA 3148 2003 (revised). http://www.osha-slc.gov/Publications/osha3148.pdf

Requirements for States and Long Term Care Facilities, 42 C.F.R. 483.13 (1992).

Requirements for States and Long Term Care Facilities, 42 C.F.R. 488.301 (1992).

Sansone, P., Schmidt, L., Nichols, J., Phillips, M., & Beslisle, S. (1998). Determining the capacity of demented nursing home residents to name a health care proxy. *Clinical Gerontologist, 19*(4), 35–50.

Strumpf, N. E., Robinson, J., Wagner, J., & Evans, L. (1998). *Restraint free care: Individualized approaches for frail elders.* New York: Springer Publishing Company.

Teno, J. M., Weitzen, S., Wetle, T., & Mor, V. (2001). Persistent pain in nursing home residents (Letter). *Journal of the American Medical Association, 285,* 2081.

Part 4

The Right to Live and the Right to Die

The success of modern medicine in preserving life has brought with it a multitude of ethical issues. The transplantation of organs has become part of the basic medical services provided in academic medical centers throughout the world. However, the procurement and allocation of organs engender a number of ethical concerns. The paradox of modern medicine is that treatment intended to save a life often ends up prolonging dying. The ethical issues of withholding and withdrawing therapy, physician-assisted suicide, persistent vegetative state, and terminal sedation are just a few of the issues addressed by the authors in chapters 14 through 16.

Chapter 14

Ethical Issues in Organ Transplantation

Carolyn H. McGrory and Linda Wright

1. What are the ethical issues in organ transplantation?

Organ transplantation is an established, lifesaving procedure that involves ethical issues around declarations of death, organ procurement issues, and the allocation of scarce societal resources, namely organs for transplantation. Declarations of death are not universally accepted, reflecting different cultural beliefs and values. The allocation of organs generally respects the principle of justice, whereby we treat like cases alike and distribute goods according to need. This is mixed with utilitarianism that requires that transplanted organs be distributed to maximize their benefit. The continuing shortage of organs for transplantation has contributed to consideration of paid donation and alternative means of procuring consent for organ donation, such as first person and presumed consent. The living donor pool now includes donors and recipients whose relationship may not be close, as well as non-directed donors and kidney transplant exchange programs. The ethical issues of voluntariness and confidentiality and the need for a balance of risks and benefits that is favorable to the living donor are significant in these developments.

The ethical issues are divided into the following categories:

- Definitions of death, which are required for organ retrieval to occur.

- The procurement of organs. This includes respect for the donor and donor family with the goal of maximizing the number of organs available for transplantation.

- The allocation of organs. This addresses both utilitarian arguments that organs should be given to those who are likely to gain maximum benefit and issues of distributive justice that suggest they should be given to those who need them most (i.e., the sickest).

2. How can those who choose to be organ donors be assured that their wishes will be followed? Who ultimately has the right to make this decision?

The autonomy of the potential donor should be respected. Some people have made their wish to be an organ donor known, either in a document such as a driver's license or by expressing their intention verbally. Family members, however, may not be aware of the individual's plan to donate. The law does not require family consent; however, hospitals are reluctant to go against a family's wishes and will approach families to obtain permission to procure organs. By knowing their loved one's previously expressed wishes, families can make a decision regarding donation, which reflects the donor's own wishes. This is within the requirements of acting as a substitute decision maker (SDM) where the SDM is charged with making the decision that he/she believes the person would have made, rather than following his/her own wishes. It is important for families to discuss these matters and know each other's wishes.

3. Is there an internationally accepted definition of death?

While the Dead Donor Rule states organ donors must be declared dead before organs may be removed, there is no one internationally accepted definition of death. Organ retrieval for transplantation requires that we be clear as to when a person is dead or alive. In the United States, the Uniform Declaration of Death Act of 1981 says, "An individual who has sustained either (1) irreversible cessation of circulatory and respiratory functions, or (2) irreversible cessation of all functions of the entire brain, including the brain stem, is dead. A determination of death must be made in accordance with accepted medical standards." This definition has been debated for some time with reference to the conflicting interests of the organ procurers and the persons who are being declared dead.

4. Is it ethical to ask a family to donate a loved one's organs when they have just been traumatized by the potential donor's death?

It is ethically acceptable provided it is done in a sensitive manner that is not harmful to the family. If the potential donor wanted to donate, we have a responsibility to try to honor that wish. Informing the family is an essential part of this. In addition, family members have the right to know that organ donation is an option they may wish to pursue. Steps on how to approach families with sensitivity are listed below.

Hospital personnel and those from the Organ Procurement Organization should establish a coordinated and uniform front. Having previously agreed on the following can help:

1. Give families a comfortable, private space in which to be together.

2. Identify the next of kin and substitute decision maker(s).

3. Allow them to spend as much time as possible with the body of their loved one.

4. Separate the act of informing them that death has occurred from the request for donation.

5. Establish a non-judgmental atmosphere that respects both donation and non-donation.

6. Provide as much counseling and support as needed. Answer questions, provide information slowly, repeat if necessary.

7. Give families adequate time to absorb information.

8. Ensure that interventions are sensitive to cultural and spiritual beliefs and practices.

9. Allow families to make their own decision without pressure to donate.

5. When there is such a shortage of organs for transplantation, why is it considered unethical and even illegal in most societies to buy an organ from a willing donor?

Arguments against legitimizing the sale of human organs include the following:

1. Selling organs is disrespectful to the sanctity of life.

2. Selling an organ would further disadvantage the poor and favor the rich.

3. People would be more vulnerable to being coerced into selling their organs.

4. Recipients may be harmed by a reduced "quality" of the organ. Persons in financial need may not have had access to appropriate health care in the past and may not disclose their entire health history.

5. Payment for organs would reduce the number of altruistic organ donations.

6. If a person buys an organ abroad and can pay for the surgery, could he/she be denied medical treatment when they return home? Will he/she be prosecuted?

The laws of the country where the sale takes place will apply to that country. Patients who have received a transplant with an organ purchased in another country will not be prosecuted on return home to the United States or Canada because they have not broken any laws that apply there. They are still eligible for posttransplant treatment according to the healthcare coverage that they have. Healthcare professionals have a duty to treat, which is enshrined in their professional codes of ethics.

7. Is there an impartial process by which the selection of candidates for transplantation is made? What are the key ethical issues we face in determining who deserves to receive an organ from the limited supply available?

Medical need, tissue matching, and length of time on the list determine the allocation of organs. Sometimes an organ is not a good match for the sickest person or the one who has waited the longest. In this case, it may be offered to a patient who has been on the list a shorter length of time because that person is the best match for the organ. A tension exists between distributive justice that would argue for the sickest candidates (whose health status may be so poor that they might die even with the newly transplanted organ) and utilitarianism that would support giving the organ to the candidate who is likely to receive the most benefit by sustaining the organ for an optimum amount of time. Candidates once denied a place on the list are now being considered for transplantation if they meet the medical and psychosocial criteria for listing (e.g., elderly patients and persons with HIV). In order to ensure equity in organ distribution, organ allocation organizations should make their methods of distributing organs transparent to the public who provide them. The transplant waiting list is national and maintained by a nonprofit organization, the United Network for Organ Sharing (UNOS), under contract to the US Department of Health and Human Services.

8. Is it ethical to use organs that may be compromised in some way?

In recent years, attempts have been made to increase the number of organs for transplantation by including organs that previously would not have been used, such as organs from older donors, from individuals with a history of hypertension or diabetes, from someone who died of a CVA or a cardiac death, someone whose kidneys had some histological abnormalities or a modest reduction in function, an individual who may have been at risk for transmitting infectious disease, or someone with malignancy. Research has shown that many of these organs function better than had previously been believed. Using these organs provides more outcomes that are more positive for many recipients than waiting on the list. The key ethical issue here is one of informed consent. A potential recipient should be informed of the likelihood of the success of transplantation with the organ that is being offered and the risks and benefits of accepting this organ or waiting for another. A recipient should not be offered an organ that is unlikely to function well and should be informed of past results of using expanded criteria organs.

9. When a family member refuses to consider donation, what are the ethical issues?

Donation is an act of beneficence; not donating is not an act of maleficence. We need to honor the autonomy of all and respect each person's freedom to choose. Organ donation is one very important way of helping someone in need, but it is not the only way and it is not for everyone. Transplantation centers should maintain a non-judgmental attitude toward those who do not offer to donate. A non-donor is entitled to make a decision that is right for him/her. The role of transplant professionals is to provide information on organ donation. It is neither to persuade nor to dissuade, but to respect a family member's wishes. Healthcare professionals should help non-donors deal with their decision not to donate and help recipients cope with their feelings toward family members who do not offer to donate.

10. Should healthcare workers approach patients' family members to consider living organ donation when the patient is reluctant to ask?

Many people say they will never ask another human being to donate an organ. Parents often have difficulty accepting an organ from an adult child.

The role of the transplant center is to educate and facilitate, but not to persuade or manipulate. Healthcare professionals should assist family members in arriving at the best decisions for them at this particular time. We do this by helping family members consider how other family members will feel, the financial and occupational consequences of donation, as well as loss of income and time away from work. It is not appropriate for healthcare professionals to ask family members directly to donate. Transplant professionals can help by making information on organ donation available to families so that the recipient does not have this responsibility. This could be in many forms, including information booklets and educational sessions. Second, they can review with potential recipients their own concerns about having someone near to them donate and help them address these issues. The final decision on approaching a potential living donor lies with the potential recipient.

11. What are the ethical challenges for the donor and for the recipient of an organ from a living donor when the organ is failing?

When the donated kidney fails to function well, recipients sometimes find it difficult to inform the donors of this and express a sense of failure and of "letting the donor down." It is important for transplant professionals to talk to recipients about this and to review with them the reasons for the failure of the graft. Recipients may need help in how to tell the donor when an organ is failing or may ask health professionals to do it for them. Donors often want to know the result of their donation and may feel some responsibility for the failing graft. Recipients and donors both need to be reminded that the outcomes of donation are not entirely predictable. Donors should be informed that there might be physiological and medical reasons for the failure.

12. Is it ethically acceptable for a stranger to donate an organ to someone in need?

The ethics of organ donation from living donors rests on the balance of risks and benefits for the donor and on the process of informed consent by which the potential donor is fully aware of those risks and benefits. It is vital that the donor's expectations of donation be realistic. The donor's motivation should be one of altruism (i.e., the wish to help someone in need of an organ without other benefit to him/herself). Organ donation from a

"Good Samaritan" may be the purest form of altruism, as a stranger is unlikely to receive any benefit other than knowing that he/she has helped someone else regain better health and achieve other life goals, such as returning to work, better function, a longer life, and resumption of a more active lifestyle. In the absence of the psychological ties between donors and recipients who know each other, strangers are accepted as organ donors when they meet medical and psychosocial criteria, and are fully informed and competent to give informed consent for the donation in question. It is illegal for a living donor to receive material goods in exchange for an organ.

13. Is it ethical to give an organ to someone whose illness is the result of chemical dependency?

Organs are distributed based on the allocation formula already outlined, not on judging past behavior. Potential recipients must meet the criteria for listing, which will include the requirement that they are no longer addicted to alcohol or illicit substances.

14. *Case:* A patient has just admitted that she is listed here and in another Organ Procurement Organization (OPO). Is this double listing ethical and/or legal?

In the United States, the candidate for an organ transplant must be placed on a local waiting list maintained by an official organ procurement organization (OPO) and on the national United Network for Organ Sharing (UNOS) waiting list to be considered. Patients may not be listed on more than one local list but may be listed in another OPO district. Others going through the waiting process may regard this double listing as questionable and even unfair, but it is legal.

15. Is it ethical to give organ transplants to people who may not have the resources to sustain them?

The cost of medications to maintain transplants can be staggering and can be up to $20,000 per year. In the United States, in the case of kidney transplants, Medicare pays for the transplant procedure and up to 44 months of medications, at which time insurance must take over or the recipients themselves must pay. By denying organs to those who have less money we would be further penalizing the financially disadvantaged. It is the responsibility of the transplant center to educate recipients about the optimum ways to care for the graft and to help them find resources to assist them. Insurers can only be held to the terms of their contracts.

16. *Case:* A post-transplant patient wants to meet her cadaveric donor's family. What are the ethical issues involved in trying to make this possible?

The wishes of both the recipient and the donor family should be respected. If either party does not wish to make contact, this wish must prevail. If both request the contact, be facilitated. Some jurisdictions discourage or ban contact while others are engaged in making this possible. If both parties wish to meet, it is important that their expectations of contact are clear and realistic. Transplant professionals can be helpful in preparing recipients and donor families for such meetings and for the feelings that may ensue.

17. Do transplant recipients have the right to bring a child into the world when they know they may be chronically ill or may die before the child is grown?

Recipients desiring pregnancy should carefully consider the advisability of becoming pregnant. The best outcome for mother, child, and graft will occur if the recipient is at optimum health at conception and this is maintained throughout the pregnancy. The concern that the viability of the graft will be affected by pregnancy can be largely allayed: in most cases, pregnancy does not adversely affect graft status. Graft loss may occur at any time unrelated to pregnancy. Recipients must consider the possibility of bringing a child into a family where it may not have a healthy or live parent to care for it. Children of transplant recipients are often premature and have a low birth weight; however, at follow-up, research indicates they are generally healthy and developing well. Ultimately, only she and her family can make the right decision for themselves.

18. If a post-transplant patient becomes pregnant, what are the ethical implications?

Pre-pregnancy counseling is the responsibility of the health professional during the initial pre-transplant patient interviews and educational sessions, as a return to fertility is a very real possibility after transplantation. Since a significant amount of time may have elapsed between these information sessions and the actual transplant, healthcare workers have an ethical responsibility to reinforce the possibility of a return to fertility and the need for contraception and careful planning in this high-risk group. With the advent of more positive post-transplant pregnancy outcomes due to the development of better immunosuppressive drugs and advances in current medical practice, the need to advise a therapeutic termination is rare, although close surveillance, with integrated care among health professionals, is necessary. In addition, genetic counseling should be recommended when a genetic impairment in the mother has been the cause for the transplant.

19. Should animals be used to grow organs for transplantation into humans? What are the ethical concerns?

Xenotransplantation, or transplants from animals, could yield an unending supply of organs, negating the need for human organ transplants. In the laboratory, most attempts at cross-species transplants have caused hyperacute rejections. Genetic modification of miniature pigs has recently been achieved, however, to make their cells more compatible for potential transplantation into humans, so this process may be more likely to succeed. Animal to human transplants are fraught with ethical dilemmas. Animal rights activists would consider that creating animals for the sole purpose of enhancing human lives is unethical. Will the recipient be a 'guinea pig' for research? Will informed consent really convey the reality of the procedure and subsequent risks? What would happen if an animal-based microbial infection were to become unleashed in the human population? At present, this mode of organ retrieval is considered highly unlikely, because of both the extreme technical nature of bringing it about and the ethical questions inherent in it.

RESOURCES

Beauchamp, T. L., & Childress, J. F. (2002). *Principles of biomedical ethics*. London: Oxford University Press.

Cupples, S. A., & Ohler, L. (Eds.). (2002). *Solid organ transplantation*. New York: Springer Publishing Company.

Lock, M. (2002). *Twice dead*. Berkeley, CA: University of California Press.

National Kidney Foundation. www.kidney.org

United Network for Organ Sharing. www.unos.org

Veatch, R. M. (2000). *Transplantation ethics*. Washington, DC: Georgetown University Press.

Chapter 15

End-of-Life Ethical Issues

JoAnne Reifsnyder, Vicki D. Lachman, Terri L. Maxwell,
Margaret M. Mahon, Catherine S. Taylor,
Sally J. Nunn, and Ursula H. Capewell

1. What are the ethical issues a clinician must confront in death and dying?

Because medical technology has become more advanced, many people expect everything to be cured. We very often believe there is something else that can and should be done. Therefore, the ethical issues at end of life have to do with three major areas: prognostication, limiting certain treatments, and appropriate roles in decision making.

Prognostication sounds simple. There are many tools to assist in decision making (e.g., APACHE, Karnovsky Performance Scale), yet patients are still too rarely given accurate data, even when physicians are provided data on a daily basis (Phillips, Hamel, Covinsky, & Lynn, 2000). Ethically, patients and families have a right to these data, and providers, patients, and families must be specific. Not, "what do you want us to do?" rather, a delineation of pathophysiology, medical indications, and then a consideration of patient preferences in that context.

This leads to the second dimension in ethical considerations in end-of-life care. Healthcare providers have a responsibility to offer treatments that can benefit patients and not to offer treatments that cannot benefit patients. This means certain treatments should not be offered. The most drastic example, and perhaps the most common, is the use of CPR. As is discussed in this chapter, CPR is often not indicated for dying patients. In fact, the burdens of CPR are not insignificant. Yet these burdens are rarely conveyed to patients and families, except when providers are trying to scare patients/families into not requesting CPR. The same guidelines apply to assisted nutrition and hydration. While tube feedings can benefit many patients, when a patient is dying or has dementia, the burdens (physiologic and otherwise) outweigh the benefits. Healthcare providers must be willing to limit technologies that are provided to dying patients.

The third dimension of ethics in end-of-life care: optimal decision-making processes. Jonsen, Siegler, and Winslade (2002) have delineated four dimensions of healthcare decision making, and the process of integrating ethics: medical indications, patient preferences, quality of life, and contextual features. In end-of-life decision making, the choices for patients, families, and healthcare providers are not endless. More specifically, respecting a patient's autonomy does not impose a duty on providers. Providers do not have to implement a therapy just because a family demands it. That is, respect for a patient's or family's autonomy exists only in the context of accurate pathophysiologic parameters. Medical indications come first.

2. What are some ways to get closure when you have experienced multiple deaths?

Multiple deaths tax one's ability to cope with loss. The question is "How do we resolve our grief when we are repeatedly affected by loss through death?" Closure means coming to terms with this loss, or figuring out what place those who have died will have in the survivors' lives.

Methods that can be helpful include the following:

1. Talk with a friend or patient's family about the importance of this patient to you. You will learn who really listens.

2. Write in your journal about the individual, including what you learned from caring for this patient and family.

3. Pray for guidance in how to let go of the individual who has affected your life, or use whatever spiritual or religious supports that help you.

4. Attend a viewing, memorial service, or funeral.

5. Build on the coping mechanisms that have helped you in the past.

6. Figure out how you want to memorialize this person, whether with pictures or poems or just internally.

3. How can I be present for dying patients without detaching from them emotionally?

When working with dying patients, it is important to know how you feel about death and dying. Our personal feelings/fears affect or even impede our ability to help patients and their families. A workshop or guided learning process can help in using personal experiences to help patients better. There may be some patients or certain times in your life when you are not able to participate fully in a patient's care. Your ability to recognize these times and make appropriate arrangements for others to do the care is essential in maintaining your well-being. Nurses should practice good health habits and seek ways to refresh themselves from the stresses of the health-care environment.

On a professional level, being knowledgeable about palliative care and applying clinical knowledge and standards to the patient care setting will give you a framework and strategies to work with the dying patient. To help the dying patient, nurses must take care of the patient's physical, emotional, and spiritual needs in a manner that is meaningful to the patient. Combining professional knowledge, personal insight, and caring should prepare the nurse to meet the challenges of this patient group.

4. What should I do when a physician gives a patient false hope?

First, when possible, have a discussion with the physician to clarify differences in perspectives to be sure you both have all the information needed to provide the patient or surrogate with optimal decision-making options. It is possible that the patient will have relegated medical decisions to family or friend in keeping with religious or cultural values (i.e., "don't ever tell me if I have cancer" or the family requests the patient not know "the truth" believing the patient will lose hope). If you continue to believe the physician is not communicating an accurate diagnosis or prognosis, or is misleading or coercive, report your concerns to the charge nurse, unit manager, and/or the ethics committee. You are a crucial advocate and have a professional responsibility to make certain that accurate information is given in a timely and appropriate manner to patients.

5.   What can I do to break through denial of impending death in a caring way?

Denial can be a therapeutic mechanism that allows individuals to get through short-term crises. As a long-term strategy, denial stops people from dealing with the reality, as painful as it may be. Patients make a great effort to maintain the possibility of a future and sometimes use denial for this purpose. Researchers have described that patients regret their role in colluding with others in not discussing their dying, once they realize that the optimism that once sustained them was just an illusion. This false optimism also hinders the patient's ability to make well-thought-out treatment decisions not based upon fear. Family members echo these same regrets, perhaps more so than the patient. Patients need to live and die with their terminal condition in their own way. When dealing with a patient in denial, do not impose the truth on the patient, but instead, explore the patient's understanding of his/her illness and his/her preference for information related to his/her medical condition and prognosis. This respects the patient's autonomy and allows him/her to determine what is best for him/her in an individual manner.

6.   If I see advance directives not being followed on a patient and a PEG tube being inserted, what is my responsibility?

Healthcare professionals must assure that the patient's wishes govern medical treatment. In this example, the nurse should review the patient's advance directive and medical record to ascertain (1) the patient's wishes pertaining to tube feeding, (2) whether the patient designated a surrogate to make decisions, (3) modifications to the advance directive, and (4) the circumstances that led to the present situation. If it is clear that the patient specifically requested no tube feeding, then the nurse needs to act. Ethical action is based on an analysis of what must be done legally, what can be done clinically, and what should be done ethically. Both a family meeting and an interdisciplinary meeting will likely be necessary to clarify the patient's wishes, authority to make decisions, the right to have advance directives honored, and the family's and team's ethical obligation.

7.   When physicians avoid approaching a family with a patient who has a poor prognosis, what should I do?

The doctrine of informed consent supports the patient's right to *receive* information about his/her condition and treatment options. Patients also have the right to *limit* the amount or type of information they receive or is disclosed to others. For example, some patients may request that the physician not disclose information about prognosis to family members.

First, the nurse should scan the progress note to reveal additional details of which the nurse may be unaware. Second, the nurse can assess the family's understanding about the patient's prognosis, including (1) what they have been told, and (2) what they expect will happen, hope will happen, and fear will happen. Third, the nurse can ask the family what is most important to them, how the team can help them to realize those wishes, and if they will allow the discussion to be shared with other team members. Fourth, the nurse can address the interdisciplinary team formally or informally in a care conference or team meeting or address the physician privately.

Finally, the nurse can directly apprise the physician that the family has needs and suggest or facilitate an approach. The nurse could accompany the physician on rounds and could model communication strategies. As the family discloses their concerns, the nurse can act as a facilitator—probing for more information, clarifying questions and responses, and summarizing key points.

If the physician is unwilling or unable to provide information that a family has requested (and which the patient has authorized), the nurse should request that the physician use another team member to address the family's concerns. If the physician refuses this step, the nurse should discuss with a supervisor and formulate a plan for responding to the family's concerns. An ethics consult might be very beneficial at such an impasse.

8. What is the best way to educate families about DNR?

CPR has become a default technology. Across health care, informed consent is needed for any intervention—patients cannot be touched without their consent . . . until the end of life. Then, permission is needed *not* to touch a patient; that is, to withhold CPR. The indications for CPR are very clear, as are the contraindications. CPR is *not* indicated when death is expected, for example, in any of the chronic diseases that cause multiorgan system failure. As with any other education, discussions with patients and families should address the goals of care and what we will do to achieve those goals. The recent trend to use the phrase Do Not *Attempt* Resuscitation (DNAR) is a good entrée for discussions about the realities of CPR.

The reality is that most patients who receive CPR will not survive to leave the hospital, and of those who survive, many will have a diminished level of functioning. In certain cases, for example, metastatic cancer, the chances of the patient surviving CPR to leave the hospital approach 0%. We owe patients these data.

9. Case: A family states that the patient would not want to go through being coded, and they also state that they "can't let go" or "believe in miracles" and, therefore, want to leave the patient a full code. What should be done?

In the absence of clear instructions from the patient, we look to the family to provide guidance about who the patient was, what he/she valued, how he/she lived, and how he/she would have viewed the current situation. In a DNR discussion, open-ended statements or questions followed by probes that are more specific can help illuminate the patient's life story. If a family member says, "Dad would never want to be coded," the nurse can respond first with "Tell me more about that . . . ," and then allow the family member ample time to respond. After we have heard their concerns, we need to determine what they know about their loved one's illness, progression, and prognosis. We also need to know what they expect will happen if he is "coded" and if he is not. Having additional members of the team available in the family meeting can be extremely helpful. Clinicians should not try to dissuade families from their values with facts or ethical arguments; trying to do this will only increase tensions and their suffering.

When family members say that they "can't let go" or expect a miracle, they are communicating their anticipatory grief, their hopes, and their fears. Further, a belief in miracles is a show of faith. Multiple meetings and opportunities to reassess the situation may be necessary. Information about the ineffectiveness of CPR in very advanced illness may be helpful. Specific spiritual or religious support provided by a trained spiritual advisor who can speak to family members knowledgeably about their religious beliefs may also be helpful. Explain that no medical interventions can interfere with a miracle, including the cessation of certain medical therapies.

10. How can I help prepare families for the patient's death?

First, determine if the family understands that the patient is dying. Ask them what they know and what it means to them. Ask them who is included in the family. Support the family by answering their questions honestly, providing them with appropriate resources, and listening attentively. Refer them to appropriate community resources, such as hospice, that may help them through this time and also those that will support them after the death.

If there is time, explore ways that they might use the time remaining. It is usually not possible to "fix" difficult family relationships, but some degree of reconciliation might be reached. If the time remaining is short, help the family prioritize what can be accomplished. As difficult as this time is, it remains an opportunity for completing unfinished business.

Help the family look at multiple ways they can assist the patient in creating a legacy; perhaps a journal, letters, scrapbook, audiotape, or video detailing their role/contribution to the family or family history. Family members may want to be involved in the patient's daily care . . . combing hair, bathing, applying lotion, or feeding. This gives them a purpose and a means of honoring the patient. Encourage conversations, reading, reminiscing, and allowing each other to express the importance of their lives. Help families understand the power of presence, just being with the patient is a comfort.

11. What are the most important things I can do to help families cope with a patient's death?

In considering how to help families adapt to life without the physical presence of the person who has died, two things must be considered. First, what were the family dynamics before the dying and death? Second, what opportunities exist at present to help the family adapt? Relationship patterns are unlikely to change when someone is dying; communication styles and patterns of relating rarely change or "get fixed" during the stressful time of someone's dying, so we should not try to change that. Still, an opportunity remains. It is often helpful to suggest to patients and families that, as difficult as the situation is, there is still a chance to say things so that in the future there are fewer "I wish I had . . . " or "what ifs . . . ?" If the patient is not responsive, telling families that it is likely that the patient can still hear, and modeling by talking with the patient whenever care is being provided, can give families permission and encouragement to do the same.

In addition, most organizations have resource lists of agencies that can provide bereavement support to families. Before an organization or individual is recommended, there should be some screening of that organization or individual's expertise.

12. How can I support chemotherapy treatment when the potential/real risks of side effects significantly affect the quality of life in end stage patients?

This question contains two very different but related issues—how can I ensure the best patient care and how can I feel okay about the treatment choices. To ensure the best possible end-of-life care we must understand patients' values concerning treatment, symptom management, suffering, and other issues. For example, patients may worry that if they decline new chemotherapy, they will be abandoned and receive either no care or inferior care.

Ideally, chemotherapy in advanced disease should not be presented as an "either/or" option—either they receive chemotherapy or they receive "comfort care." Comfort care (palliative care) should be an integral part of any seriously ill patient's plan of care. The patient and family should be introduced to the concepts and goals of palliative care early. The bottom line is that the patient needs to choose, but needs adequate prognostic data to make this choice.

This question also touches on the nurse's values concerning quality of life, suffering, sacrifice, dependency, and death. Nurses need to know where they stand on issues concerning life and death. That means that sometimes nurses have to watch patients make choices that they do not think they would make under the same circumstances. When we feel conflicted about a patient's choice, we need to step back and ask ourselves, "Is this the *patient's* need or *my* need?" If we need support, then we need to take care of ourselves and find that support in colleagues.

13. *Case:* A patient's daughter has Healthcare Power of Attorney. She repeatedly states, "I know my mother wouldn't want to be kept alive on this ventilator but I can't let her die." What should I do?

If possible, find a quiet location to optimize communication and a discussion of why she feels this way. Listening is one of the most important skills that help in complex decision making, providing the agonized relative a chance to ventilate their feelings. It is important to let the daughter know she is not "letting" her mother die. Her mother's medical condition is determining whether she will live or die and honoring her mother's wishes is a difficult, but loving act. Emphasize that the decision to withhold or withdraw must be made from the patient's perspective and may not be the one the daughter would choose for herself. The daughter's role is to speak for her mother and facilitate the decision her mother would make if she could awaken from her condition and speak. Often other family members, social service, or clergy can provide support the daughter needs to deal with her grief. In some instances requesting assistance from the ethics committee, the patient representative, and/or chaplain may be necessary to help the daughter honor her mother's wishes. Some of the issues that may complicate surrogate decisions are grief, shock, angst, depression, frustration, anger, and other family dynamics. It may unburden the daughter to know that as much as what she wants matters to us, healthcare decisions must be based on what her mother wants, and her job is "merely" to convey her mother's wishes.

14. What is a persistent vegetative state (PVS)? What are the ethical issues that I am likely to confront?

Persistent vegetative state (PVS) is a condition in which severe bilateral cerebral damage (either from an acute event or as a result of progressive dementia) results in irreversible coma, leaving only autonomic functions intact. Patients in a PVS will have no awareness but sleep/wake cycles and other autonomic responses such as eye movement, swallowing, grimacing, and papillary changes in response to light may remain. The presence of these reflexes may be confusing and disturbing to onlookers, who may interpret them as evidence that the patient can respond and will recover. However, when PVS is properly diagnosed, the prognosis for recovery is highly unlikely. Because most patients with PVS can breathe on their own, ethical considerations generally center on whether or not to continue life-supporting interventions, including artificial feeding. The question arises as to whether this is "a life worth living."

Furthermore, in many cases, the wishes of the patient are not known and decisions are left to surrogates. It is important to help the surrogates recognize that patients in a vegetative state lack sensation; therefore, they cannot experience distress if a decision is made to withhold or withdraw a therapy. Decisions about medical intervention should be based on an assessment of the ratio of benefits to burdens for the patient.

15. Why does withdrawing therapy feel so different from withholding treatment?

While withdrawal of treatment and withholding of treatment are ethically indistinguishable, removing life-prolonging treatment "feels" qualitatively different both to the patient/family and to the clinician. Treatment withdrawal "feels" like something that we are doing *to* patients rather than *for* them. Not starting a treatment (withholding) engages us far less than acting to discontinue a device or treatment. We may mistakenly believe that the act of following the patient's wishes will be the proximate cause of death. In fact, continuing technological means to sustain can impose enormous suffering and do little to prevent the inevitable.

Three ideas may permit the nurse to feel differently about treatment withdrawal. First, withdrawing interventions that the patient deems burdensome is an act of compassion. Second, life-sustaining treatment such as artificial nutrition/hydration may not prolong life. Recent studies demonstrate little or no difference in survival for patients who receive such treatments at the end of life and those who do not. Third, a "trial" of treatment followed by withdrawal is arguably a stronger ethical stance—discontinuation in that case will be based on evidence about the efficacy and desirability of the intervention.

16. What are the official criteria for brain death? How can I explain this to the family?

With the advent of technology such as mechanical ventilators that can breathe for a person who has lost brainstem function, it became clear that a new determination of death was needed to replace the "cardio-respiratory criterion" of death. In 1981, the Uniform Definition of Death (UDDA) proposed a new definition of death. A person is now considered dead if he/she has sustained either irreversible cessation of circulatory or respiratory function, or irreversible cessation of all functions of the entire brain, including the brain stem. Brain death is further determined by:

1. unresponsiveness to intensely painful stimuli;

2. no movements or breathing for a period of at least 1 hour or if on a ventilator, 3 or more minutes without spontaneous breathing if the respirator is turned off;

3. no reflexes; and

4. a flat electroencephalogram (EEG) recorded for a minimum of 10 minutes and repeated at least 24 hours later with no change.

Since no medical goals can be attained for someone who is dead, all interventions should be terminated. Families should be informed of their loved one's death in a sensitive manner; however, there is no ethical or legal requirement to gain permission of the family to discontinue therapy in a brain dead person.

17. **Case: A patient's husband wants to take his wife off the respirator and he has asked the physician to write a DNR order. Her son and I have both had conversations with her where she has stated she wants to live. What should I do if there is a code?**

Questions about DNR orders are best answered by considering the following:

1. the likelihood of success (i.e., would resuscitation succeed and would the patient be likely to be discharged from the hospital?),

2. the known preferences of the patient, and

3. the expected quality of life of the patient if resuscitation succeeds.

In the case where a patient has expressed the wish to live but a family member has decided to remove life-sustaining therapy and requested a DNR order, the wishes of the patient need to be advocated. However, an expression of "wanting to live" does not necessarily mean that the patient would have wanted treatment continued if the treatment is believed to be futile. Perhaps the husband understands that although his wife wants to live, she would not like to live in her present condition if there were no hope for recovery. The nurse should advocate for an emergency family meeting to explore these issues and perhaps request an ethics committee consultation to assist in the matter.

18. **Case: A physician wants to do a trial intervention of ventilator support for a patient recuperating from aneurysm surgery because she has now developed pneumonia. The family is afraid that the patient will be "held hostage" by technology. What could I say to reassure the family?**

Family members are the proxy decision makers and, therefore, should be making decisions that the patient would be

making. Help them determine what that "substituted judgment" would be. Reassure the family that trial interventions
are discontinued if they are unsuccessful. Work with the appropriate medical teams to ensure that a time for the trial is
specified and will be followed. Help the family understand
that there is no difference between withdrawing and withholding of treatment.

19. *Case:* **A patient is clearly dying, but the physician refuses to refer him to hospice. What is my ethical responsibility?**

While hospice may be the ideal for many patients approaching the end of life, the nurse's *ethical* responsibility to
the dying patient does not necessarily demand a hospice referral. The nurse's obligation to promote comfort and relieve pain can still be met in a non-hospice setting for care.
On the other hand, the nurse's responsibilities to safeguard
the patient's welfare and to intervene when unethical conduct is observed could be construed as an ethical mandate
to act when the patient is denied hospice access.

If the physician refuses to refer the hospice-eligible patient, the nurse should discuss the situation directly with the
physician. If the patient desires and is eligible for hospice
care, then he/she is entitled to receive such care, and the
nurse should work through the appropriate institutional channels to ensure that the patient's rights are upheld. While it is
possible for the patient who desires hospice to self-refer
and/or to locate another physician who will refer, pursuing
one of these paths *without* addressing the issue of the physician who is obstructing patient access to an entitlement simply circumvents a serious problem—one that is not likely to
resolve on its own.

20. **If a chronically ill patient does not have an advance
directive, how can I help them complete a Living Will/
Healthcare Power of Attorney or other type of advance directive?**

Tell them that you share this information with all patients as part of excellent
care. Advance directives should be viewed as a loving act. It is an opportunity
for patients to express the healthcare choices that they desire based on

their values. When this information is shared with families and healthcare providers, difficult decisions can be made with the assurance that this is what the person would want. You might use a personal story to illustrate how sharing this information lifts some of the family's burden and allows them to proceed with their grief work.

Information about advance directives should be given in a sequential fashion moving at the patient's pace. It begins with a discussion of what the patient's values are and ends with the desires being documented. Using written information and/or videos to supplement and clarify the conversations is very effective. These conversations take time and other resources can be used as needed. Explore concerns about the process involving other members of the healthcare team as appropriate, such as patient advocates. Knowing that advance directives take effect only when the person cannot speak for him/herself and that they can be revoked at any time the person is competent provides reassurance that patients have control over their choices.

Finally, a formal document is not necessary. If the team understands the patient's wishes, and whom the patient designates to represent his/her wishes in decision making, then the goal has been met in a way often less threatening to patients.

RESOURCES

American Academy of Hospice and Palliative Medicine. www.aahpm.org

American College of Physicians. Papers by End-of-Life Care Consensus Panel. www.acponline.org/letters/papers.htm

American Nurses Association. (2001). *Code of ethics for nurses with interpretive statements*. Washington, DC: American Nurses Publishing.

Center to Advance Palliative Care. www.cape.org

Center for Ethics in Health Care (Oregon Health & Science University). "Ethics and End-of-Life Care Links of Interest." An exhaustive list of links related to ethics and end-of-life care. www.ohsu.edu/ethics/links.htm

Center for Palliative Care Education (University of Washington). "Advanced Care Planning Articles." http://depts.washington.edu/pallcare/resources.php?category =3

Colm, L., Doyle, R. L., & Raffin, R. A. (1999). Do-not-resuscitate orders in the face of patient and family opposition. *Critical Care Medicine, 27*, 1045–1047.

ELNEC: End-of-Life Nursing Education Consortium. (2000). Supported by Robert Wood Johnson Foundation. Princeton, NJ: American Association of Colleges of Nursing, City of Hope, and the ELNEC project team.

Ferrell, B. R., & Coyle, N. (Eds.). (2005). *Textbook of palliative nursing*. New York: Oxford University Press.

Hospice and Palliative Care Nurses Association. www.hpna.org

Jonsen, A. R., Siegler, M., & Winslade, W. J. (2002). *Clinical ethics: A practical approach to ethical decisions in clinical medicine* (5th ed.). New York: McGraw-Hill.

Lynn, J., & Harrold, J. (1999). *Handbook for mortals: Guidance for people facing serious illness*. New York: Oxford University Press.

Massachusetts General Hospital Stroke Service. "Determination of Death Using Brain Criteria." Retrieved May 31, 2005, http://neuro-oas.mgh.harvard.edu/stop stroke/brain_death.htm

National Hospice and Palliative Care Association. Has excellent information on advance care planning. www.caringinfo.org

Panke, J. T., & Coyne, P. (2004). *Conversations in palliative care*. Pensacola, FL: Pohl Publishing, Inc.

Phillips, R. S., Hamel, M. B., Covinsky, K. E., & Lynn, J. (2000). Findings from SUPPORT and HELP: an introduction. Study to understand prognoses and preferences for outcomes and risks of treatment. Hospitalized elderly longitudinal project. *Journal of the American Geriatrics Society, 48 (5 Suppl)*, S1–5.

Webb, M. (1997). *The good death: The new American search to reshape the end of life*. New York: Bantam Books.

Chapter 16

The Right to Die: Ethical Issues

Sally J. Nunn, Vicki D. Lachman, Margaret M. Mahon,
Catherine S. Taylor, Terri L. Maxwell,
Ursula H. Capewell, and JoAnne Reifsnyder

1. What are key ethical principles in caring for the dying patient?

Some of the more common ethical principles used when exploring decisions for the dying patient are

1. autonomy

2. non-maleficence/beneficence

3. truth telling

4. professional/patient relationship

Ethical principles usually hold one to a higher standard than legal principles.

Principle of autonomy supports the self-determination of a dying patient. For example, in order to make an informed decision, a person must understand the choice and consequences of a chemotherapy or radical surgery choice. Adequate information about one's diagnosis and prognosis needs to be presented in a way that is understandable to the person. When it is assessed that a person is not able to make choices, then a surrogate decision maker is identified either through advance directives or next of kin.

"First do no harm" is derived from the principle of non-maleficence/ beneficence. Healthcare providers are obligated not to intentionally inflict harm, strive to prevent harm, remove harm, and promote good. This principle may be applied to decisions regarding withholding and withdrawing life sustaining treatment or weighing benefits versus burdens.

Truth telling also supports the doctrine of informed consent. The patient may not want information about a procedure, choosing instead to defer to a family member to give consent. Truth telling is essential to developing a trusting relationship between the dying patient and the nurse.

The professional/patient relationship is based on the above principles as well as privacy, confidentiality, and fidelity. Guidelines for this relationship are in the *Code of Ethics for Nurses*. Most nurses assume the role of patient advocate, which entails acting in the patient's best interest. However, this might not always coincide with the nurse's beliefs resulting in conflict, such as patient's desire for physician-assisted suicide. The remaining questions and answers are designed to help the nurse negotiate a solution to difficult ethical situations.

2. How can I increase my comfort level with increasing the opioid dose for pain management?

The most common fear about using opioids is that too much will kill the patient. First, physiologically—titrating *to symptoms* will not hasten death. The goal of palliative care is optimum symptom management across disease trajectories. Unfounded fears not uncommonly interfere with provision of optimal care. Just as we should give appropriate antihypertensive or insulin for hypertension or diabetes, so, too, we must provide appropriate medications, including opioids, for the management of pain and dyspnea.

Second, many people will call upon the doctrine of double effect in this circumstance. This doctrine, first written by Thomas Aquinas in the Middle Ages and expounded on by many since that time, is complex and subtle. The four conditions of the doctrine, which recognizes that some actions can have good and bad effects, are:

1. the intended act must be good or neutral;

2. the good effect must be the sole intent of the action, though the bad effect is foreseen;

3. the bad effect must not be the means to attain the good effect;

4. the good effect must outweigh the bad effect.

The reality is that the doctrine of double effect does *not* apply in most end-of-life care. Optimal symptom management rarely hastens death, including administration of opioids. Further, the doctrine of double effect does not absolve providers from responsibility for their actions; it does challenge providers to be clear and honest about their intent.

3. What is the best way to proceed when the patient clearly is terminal and suffering and the family still insists on doing everything, even after they have received much education on the issues?

Ask them what "doing everything" means to them. Explore the values and beliefs that led them to this decision. They may fear that if high-tech treatment is withdrawn then the patient will not receive care. Every aggressive measure should be taken to alleviate the patient's symptoms, addressing medical, psychological, and spiritual care. [The nurse is in a unique position to act as an advocate for the patient/family to ensure that care is provided in a way that is meaningful to them.]

Interventions or treatment that will not benefit the patient should not be provided. If the physicians cannot support the family in aggressive treatment that medically might benefit the patient, then appropriate measures should be taken to transfer care of the individual to a provider who can work with the family.

4. Why is withdrawing medically provided nutrition and hydration to a terminally ill patient not physician assisted suicide (PAS)?

Again, pathophysiology must be the first parameter that frames the options of clinical decision making. The natural trajectory of many diseases is a decrease in the patient's hunger and desire to eat. For many patients, tube feedings do not, in fact, prevent aspiration pneumonia, pressure ulcers, infection, nor do they improve functional status and especially mortality. Patients who continue to receive assisted nutrition and hydration may accumulate fluid in their lungs, and in other physiologic spaces that cause pain and discomfort without benefit. Forced fluids and nutrition often increases the burdens on the dying patient.

Very often, assisted nutrition and hydration, whether through TPN or PEG tube, are started because they *can* be started; introducing assisted feeding is taken as the default option. These are recognized as a technology that the patient can refuse, but more importantly, as procedures that are often *not* indicated in care of a patient who is dying.

It is important to note that the U.S. Supreme Court did acknowledge that patients have a right to refuse treatment. It is largely based on this that the Patient Self Determination Act was written in 1990.

5. What is my obligation to a patient when treatment and technology are prolonging the dying and care is futile?

A nurse's primary obligation is to the patient. When the nurse believes the treatment being provided is only prolonging the patient's dying and the burdens of treatment have become disproportionate to the anticipated benefits, the nurse should discuss his/her concerns with the medical team. The nurse should ask the patient's physician(s) to outline the current goals of care as well as the level of probability for attaining such goals. The nurse should also assess the patient's and/or family's understanding of the situation. In addition, the nurse can encourage the team to have an open discussion with the patient and/or family about the appropriateness of forgoing life-sustaining treatment if the goals of medicine now appear unlikely to be attainable, reassuring them that appropriate care will continue to be provided.

6. *Case:* A patient is terminally ill and has a copy of the book *Final Exit* by Derek Humphry and praises Dr. Kevorkian. What is my responsibility?

Begin with the statement "I'm interested in understanding why you admire Dr. Kevorkian." First and foremost recognize this as an opportunity for a discussion of the patient's values and fears (e.g., pain, dependency, debilitation, abandonment, loss of mental acuity). If you do not agree with the statement, at least support the patient's right to this opinion; do not enter into a debate unless the patient indicates an interest in doing so. If you are able to identify the concerns of the patient, assure him/her that you will aggressively pursue management of these concerns in any way you can, offering examples of what you intend to do if the patient agrees. Encourage him/her to complete an advance directive and a values history. Express no judgment on his/her choices but offer support and reassurance that symptom management and social support is a high priority of care. Your ultimate responsibility is to listen to the patient and consider it a positive that he/she feels secure enough to be able to express his/her thoughts to you.

7. *Case:* A patient is experiencing severe dyspnea, not relieved by oxygen, morphine, and other comfort measures. He is asking to be "put to sleep." What ethical options can I offer?

This is perhaps one of the most difficult encounters that providers can experience. The goal of care remains the same: optimal symptom management. Two steps must happen at this point: assure the patient of your continued presence (that is, you're not scared off by the request), and find out what the patient is really requesting. The majority of patients are not asking for hastened death, but are expressing a fear that their symptoms will get out of control. Reassurance of continued presence and aggressive symptom management is essential.

It is important to convey that the majority of symptoms can be managed. In those rare cases when they cannot, palliative sedation may be an option. *Palliative sedation* differs from terminal sedation in several ways; most importantly, it's reversible. The goal of palliative sedation is to alleviate distress for patients for whom other methods of symptom relief have been unsuccessful. Palliative sedation is *not* a means to hasten death, but is for managing the patient's suffering.

In June 1997, the U.S. Supreme Court unequivocally supported the patient's right to refuse treatment, even if refusing that treatment meant the patient might die sooner than with other treatments. Justices O'Connor (a breast cancer survivor) and Souter wrote powerfully about the responsibility "to alleviate that suffering, even to the point of causing unconsciousness and hastening death."

8. How does the Netherlands ethically justify euthanasia? Are people being put to death against their will there?

Until 2001, there was no "law" on the books authorizing euthanasia in the Netherlands. For decades there was a tacit agreement that physicians would not be prosecuted for assisting patients to die as long as they adhered to certain rules. The number of cases of physician-assisted suicide has increased over the years, and there are concerns that the practice is becoming acceptable for patients with chronic illnesses who are not imminently terminal, for extreme mental suffering, and in cases where the patient is not able to consent. This "slippery slope" is the assumption that a practice will become more socially acceptable over time for larger and more diverse groups of patients. The concern is that eventually it could become acceptable to put patients to death against their will. Another concern is that patients would sense a "duty to die" to spare their family members months of pain and possible financial hardship. There is conflicting evidence that patients are being put to death against their will in the Netherlands.

The support for physician-assisted suicide both here and abroad is rooted in patient autonomy. Those who support the practice maintain that individuals' sovereignty over their lives extends to the timing of their death. They further assert that only the individual himself/herself can really say when life is worth living. Without specific medical assistance to end life, the individual who wishes to die to escape an intolerable life may perceive that the only options are violent means (such as weapons or suffocation), stockpiling drugs to induce an overdose (which may or may not result in death), or attempting suicide with over-the-counter preparations (often ineffective). Recent literature (Erich, 2001) has supported voluntary refusal of food and fluids as a means to more peacefully hasten death.

9. How should I respond to a patient who requests my help in dying?

Clinicians, policy makers, and ethicists generally agree that comprehensive palliative care is the standard of care for the dying, but there are rare instances when life has become intolerable despite the best efforts to alleviate symptoms. When a nurse is confronted with a "help me die" request it is an important opportunity for an exploration of the patient's fears and concerns pertaining to the dying process. It should also prompt a thorough assessment of the adequacy of the palliative care plan and consideration of the goals of the treatments . . . do the benefits outweigh the burdens? Assure the patient you will not abandon him/her and that you will continue aggressive pursuit of comfort care measures. Other areas may be causing anxiety (e.g., financial, spiritual, family estrangement); therefore, social services, clergy, and/or the patient representative may be able to lend assistance. Encourage the patient to discuss these concerns with the attending physician.

10. Are the nurses in Oregon ethically/legally allowed to participate when a patient chooses PAS?

The Oregon Nurses' Association (ONA) Position Paper on the Death with Dignity Act discusses the nurse's role in cases where the nurse chooses to stay involved, as well as where the nurse chooses to withdraw on moral grounds.

If the patient inquires about the option of assisted suicide, the nurse is to share relevant information about this legal option. If the nurse chooses to stay involved, then the nurse's role is to provide palliative care and the following:

1. Explore reasons for the patient's request to end his/her life and make a determination as to whether the patient is depressed and whether the depression is influencing his/her decision; or whether the patient has made a rational decision based on the patient's own fundamental values and beliefs

2. Be present during the patient's self-administration of the medication and during the patient's death to console and counsel the family

The nurse may also choose on moral and ethical grounds not to be involved in the care of a patient who has chosen assisted suicide. However, the nurse must provide for the patient's safety, avoid abandonment, and withdraw only when assured that all alternative sources of care are available to the patient.

The nurse may not inject or administer the medication that will lead to the end of the patient's life (e.g., administer pills, put pills in patient's hand, or hold pills while patient takes them). The nurse who chooses not to be involved also cannot subject patients, families, peers, or other members of the healthcare team to judgmental comments on their actions because of their decision to choose or participate in assisted suicide. The ANA (2001) in the *Code of Ethics for Nurses* and a number of nurse specialty organizations' position papers include public statements against nurse participation in PAS.

11. What ethical reasons does the "right to die movement" use to support PAS and euthanasia?

With advancing disease often comes the escalation of undesirable symptoms. When symptoms become so distressing that life does not seem worth living and everything seems to be out of control then physician-assisted suicide (PAS) might be considered. Currently, adults with decision-making capacity who experience intractable suffering have a legal and ethical right to refuse, withhold, or withdraw all treatment, even when that choice will hasten their death.

The right-to-die movement supporters argue that declining, withholding, and/or withdrawing treatment are the same from a consequential perspective as PAS. They believe that PAS supports the individual's autonomy and beneficence, in that it provides the individual with a choice and relief from suffering. It is important to remember that PAS is patient initiated, without duress, and that the patient understands all of the ramifications of his/her actions.

12. How are the cases of Karen Ann Quinlan and Nancy Beth Cruzan relevant to nursing practice?

These two landmark cases set important precedents for the right to refuse unwanted medical treatment and to affirm the right of a surrogate to make decisions when the patient is unable to speak for him/herself. The Quinlan case was decided by the New Jersey Supreme Court in 1976 after prolonged and agonizing legal battles. The father petitioned the courts to allow him to remove the ventilator from his 26-year-old daughter, who was in a persistent vegetative state (PVS), saying she would want to "die with dignity." It was the first "right to die" case in the country. Some of the major findings of that decision are:

- Every competent adult has a fundamental right to privacy/liberty guaranteed under the 14th amendment to the U.S. Constitution that includes the *right to refuse medical treatment.*

- A guardian *(surrogate) may assert the right on the patient's behalf* and may render his/her best judgment as to whether the patient would terminate treatment under the circumstances, affirming the legal import of advance directives.

- There is *no valid distinction between "ordinary" and "extraordinary"* means of treatment (e.g., receiving insulin to refusing ventilator).

The Cruzan case was similar in nature (a 28-year-old in PVS). The family demanded the right to withdraw her feeding tube, stating she would never want to exist for years on machines in a condition "like Karen Quinlan." A long battle through the Missouri courts led to the only "right to die" case to be heard by the United States Supreme Court. The Court returned the case to the jurisdiction of the State, but with the following comments:

- Majority held there was *no legal distinction between removal of a ventilator and artificial nutrition*; both are medical treatment.

- Majority of the U.S. Supreme Court would find it *unconstitutional to ignore (or override) the treatment directives of a healthcare agent.*

- *No legal distinction between withdrawing and withholding* (e.g., once a treatment has been initiated it can be discontinued).

It is, therefore, important to keep in mind that the patient is in charge of his/her own body. If an adult with decision-making capacity (understands the risks, consequences and outcomes of decisions) refuses a medical treatment he/she is constitutionally protected. Second, a surrogate (proxy decision maker) has the same authority to speak on behalf of the patient who lacks capacity.

13. What is the Hemlock Society, and can I refer patients to it?

The Hemlock Society, a non-profit membership association, is the oldest and largest right-to-die organization. It consists of more than 30,000 members in all states and the District of Columbia. Members have access to programs that help them and their loved ones examine the full range of end-of-life options, including options of hastening the dying process.

The Society works through the democratic process to change the law and

1. Educates the public on advance healthcare directives, living wills, durable powers of attorney, and other resources that help ensure their end-of-life wishes are followed.

2. Provides materials for healthcare professionals and legislators.

3. Proposes legislated safeguards to protect both patients and physicians.

4. Endorses physician-assisted dying for the terminally ill *only* as a last resort and strongly endorses better pain management and universal access to hospice care.

If patients are interested in obtaining more information, they may be referred to the Hemlock Society's Web site at www.hemlock.org. A book entitled *Final Exit* (1991) by the founder of the Hemlock Society, Derek Humphry, also is available.

14. How is suffering different from pain? How can I help a patient who is suffering?

Too many care providers fail to recognize pain beyond the physical dimension. The mental aspects of pain and suffering include, but are not limited to, immobility, dependency, abandonment, spiritual anguish, and multiple disorders (e.g., blindness, hearing, loss of bowel and bladder control). Your role in identifying these concerns and facilitating modalities that will ease these concerns is crucial to providing optimal care for dying and/or chronically ill patients. Constipation, sleeplessness, and unrelenting nausea are examples of great suffering in very ill patients. Be sure to ask the patient what bothers him/her and facilitate resolution as much as possible.

15. What do we need to do first before we consider legalizing PAS and euthanasia? Does patient suffering justify them?

Suffering is presently cited as a justification for PAS and euthanasia by voluntary euthanasia societies. The rising tide of public opinion in favor of PAS and euthanasia is based on fear and lack of medical knowledge. The number of supporters also depends on which study you read and how the questions are worded.

However, comprehensive and multidisciplinary palliative care can effectively relieve most of the suffering of the terminally ill. Therefore, we need to educate nurses and physicians to deliver palliative care. All countries that have legalized PAS and euthanasia have a universal, accessible healthcare system. We would first need to protect the vulnerable citizens— the aged, the sick, the disabled, and those who feel a burden to others— experiencing pressure to request euthanasia.

16. What are the top reasons patients request PAS and what can I do to help patients?

There are a multitude of reasons why a patient may request physician-assisted suicide. The reasons frequently arise from physical, psychological, social, and or spiritual suffering making living unbearable.

Intractable pain, although frequently cited, is only one of the reasons that PAS requests are initiated. At the top of the list is the very strong sense of being a burden and dependent on others. Next on the list is the intolerance of physical disintegration; to include intractable nausea and vomiting, coughing with or without the sensation of suffocation, dyspnea, swallowing difficulties, loss of control over bodily functions (bowels and/or bladder), extreme fatigue, and depression. Depression leads to viewing life as meaningless and not worth living.

Nurses should respond to PAS requests non-judgmentally, provide all relevant information (to include alternative treatments and options), involve the multidisciplinary team to evaluate the patient's rationale for the request, help clarify the patient's goals, and, last but not least, ensure adequate management of *all* symptoms at a level acceptable to the patient and family.

17. Does Switzerland allow euthanasia to be performed by non-physicians and for non-Swiss residents? If so, how is this ethically justified?

Switzerland allows assisted suicide based on altruistic (unselfish motives) and is a country where resources for palliative care are not yet available to all terminally ill patients. Swiss law does not consider suicide a crime or assisting suicide as complicity in a crime. It views suicide as possibly rational. Switzerland's Parliament has debated decriminalizing euthanasia, but at the present it is still considered a crime. The involvement of a physician is usually considered a necessary safeguard in assisted suicide; Holland, Belgium, and the U.S. state of Oregon all require it. However, in Switzerland, Article 115 does not require the involvement of physicians, or that the patient be terminally ill; it only requires that the motive be unselfish. This reliance on a base motive, rather than on the intent to kill to define a crime, is foreign to Anglo-Saxon jurisprudence, but it is pivotal in continental Europe.

A joint statement in 2002 by the Swiss Medical Association and the Swiss Nurses' Association placed assisted suicide outside the purview of professional oversight and referred to physicians and nurses as citizens. This allows them, like other citizens, to altruistically assist suicide. All hospitals have barred assisted suicide from their premises.

Recently, the practice of a Zurich based Right to Die Society that offers assisted suicide to non-resident foreigners has attracted a great deal of media attention and concern. This could eventually result in increased regulation, but a radical departure from Switzerland's unique stance on this issue seems unlikely.

18. What can be done when family members disagree on end-of-life treatment decisions relative to an incapacitated patient?

Terri Schiavo, a young woman who was kept alive in a PVS for 15 years by being fed artificially through a PEG tube, is a tragic example of the decisions families must make when technological advances prolong a life some might view as "not worth living." This Florida case represents the tragedy of a family divided (husband versus parents) on who should decide on behalf of an incapacitated loved one. Most similar conflicts can and should be decided as close to the bedside as possible, not in the glare of national headlines with legal and political wrangling. Communication clarification, usually through provision of a family forum and often arranged by the unit manager, ethics committee, or patient advocate, is the most effective way to diffuse escalating emotions and avoid the most invasive process of decision making by strangers (the courts, guardians, judges, and lawyers). Listening closely to the dissenting voices cannot be overrated and is an effective tool in conflict resolution.

19. The Oregon-based organization, Compassion in Dying, helps people not die alone. What else should nurses know about it?

Compassion in Dying provides information, consultation, and emotional support to individuals for all end-of-life choices. Compassion in Dying has been on the forefront of providing support to individuals who choose physician-assisted suicide as part of Oregon's Death with Dignity Act. Compassion encourages eligible patients to contact the organization in the early stages of their illness, so that they can establish an ongoing relationship to adequately explore the full range of options to relieve suffering and discuss other end-of-life issues. The organization also offers publications such as *Dying Right: The Death With Dignity Movement* and *Compassion in Dying, Stories of Dignity and Choice*.

The organization's legal advocacy made front page news in *Oregon v. Ashcroft*. The organization successfully fought "Ashcroft Directive," which attempted to override the option of dispensing controlled substances for the legitimate purpose of assisting suicide. It ruled that physicians and pharmacists are immune from civil and criminal liability or any adverse disciplinary action for participating in good faith compliance with the Oregon Act.

20. The Bergman versus Chin case set a precedent on pain management. What conclusion did this case reach that is relevant to nursing practice?

Edward Bergman was an 85-year-old patient at the Eden Medical Center in Castro Valley, California, in February 1998. His probable diagnosis was lung cancer. Dr. Wing Chin, an internist, was Mr. Bergman's physician. Mr. Bergman's family sued Dr. Chin, claiming that Dr. Chin inadequately managed Mr. Bergman's pain, and this was a form of elder abuse (*Bergman v. Eden Medical Center*, No. H205732-1). Dr. Chin said that he ordered the doses of medication that he did (25 mg meperidine, and later, a fentanyl patch) because he did not want to cause Mr. Bergman's death. Further, Chin claimed that the lung cancer was never proven, and that he was treating compression fracture pain. Chin claimed that the medications and every 2-hour turning that he ordered were appropriate management for compression fracture. The jury awarded $1.5 million to Bergman's family; the case was later settled for $375,000.

The case is significant for two reasons. It has received widespread attention because it is believed to have set a standard for adequate pain management. Less widely cited is the fact that this was the first case in which the California Elder Abuse statutes resulted in a verdict against a physician.

RESOURCES

Beauchamp, T. L., & Childress, J. F. (2001). *Principles of biomedical ethics*. New York: Oxford University Press.
Compassion in Dying Federation. http://www.compassionindying.org
Erich, L. (2001). Terminal sedation, self-starvation and orchestrating the end of life. *Archives of Internal Medicine, 62*(3), 329–332.
The Hemlock Society. http://www.hemlock.org
Humphry, D. (1991). *Final exit: The practicalities of self-deliverance and assisted suicide for the dying*. New York: Dell Publishing.
International Task Force on Euthanasia and Assisted Suicide. http://www.inter nationaltaskforce.org

Kerkhof, A. J. (2000). How to deal with requests for assisted suicide: Some experiences and practical guidelines from the Netherlands. *Psychology, Public Policy & Law, 6*(2), 452–466.

Oregon Nurses Association. http://www.oregonrn.org/services-whitepapers-000.php

Quill, T. E., Dresser, R., & Brock, D. W. (1997). The rule of double effect—a critique of its role in end-of-life decision making. *New England Journal of Medicine, 337*(24), 1768–1771.

Snyder, L., & Caplan, A. (Eds.). (2002). *Assisted suicide: Finding common ground.* Bloomington, IN: Indiana University Press.

Spiro, H. M., Curnen, M. G., & Wandel, L. P. (Eds.). (1996). *Facing death: Where culture, religion, and medicine meet.* New Haven, CT: Yale University Press.

Troy, T. New type of suit: Pain treatment. *National Law Journal.* http://www.law.washington.edu/courses/mastroianni/B505

Part 5

Developing an Organizational Culture That Supports Ethical Behavior

The Joint Commission on Accreditation Healthcare Organizations (JCAHO) recognizes the need for organizational support for ethical behavior in its standards. JCAHO 2005 "Ethics, Rights and Responsibility Standards for Hospitals" covers 25 expectations for ethical organization. For example, one standard states "The organization follows ethical behavior in its care, treatment, services and business practices."

Part 5 begins with the organization's relationship to managed care and ends with the important contribution that ethics committees make to supporting ethical practice. Organizational, leadership, and labor ethics chapters focus on the important role leaders, at all levels, in the organization play in creating an ethical environment. Actions do speak louder than policies and procedures.

Chapter 17

Access to Care and Ethical Issues

Caroline Camuñas

1. Does everyone have a right to health care?

When uninsured people go to an emergency room with an emergency condition, they must receive care if the organization receives Federal funds. Medicare and Medicaid provide Federal funds to all healthcare organizations.

It is very difficult to justify a right to health care, because in doing so you ask others to do something. You cannot have a right unless there is a duty or obligation to meet that right. There is no constitutional amendment specific to health and health care. Rights language may be used to emphasize areas where social change is needed to form a more just system.

2. *Case:* An elderly patient is going to have surgery. Since this patient is old, wouldn't it be better to use the funds on someone younger and just let the old patient die?

Decisions on rationing of health care should not be made at a particular patient's expense. Denying treatment based on age, religion, gender, or ethnicity is unethical as well as illegal. If the treatment is useful, it should be done. Treatment can often make it easier to provide care, ease pain and suffer-

223

ing, and, in the long run, save money as well as improve quality of life.

3. Why must we get approval from the health maintenance organization (HMO) to do a clearly needed test on a patient?

Approvals must be obtained in an effort to control costs. There have always been gatekeepers for health care. In the past, the gatekeepers were health-care professionals. The shift to managed care has added administrative costs and more decision makers, which, in turn, increases professional moral distress as well as consumes valuable time.

4. If a patient has a do not resuscitate (DNR) order, why do we continue to spend money to treat him or her?

A DNR order is just that: if the patient has a cardiac arrest, nothing further is to be done. There is nothing to suggest that care and treatment stop. Indeed, we must provide care. This obligation is included in the American Nurses Association (2001) *Code of Ethics for Nurses* and states "The nurse promotes, advocates for, and strives to protect the health, safety, and rights of the patient" (p. 12).

5. What are the potential compromises of managed care?

The unavoidable issues and challenges of managed care are:

1. tension between cost containment and quality of care,

2. threats to the patient-professional relationship,

3. policies that constrain professional judgment,

4. safeguarding patients from harm,

5. allocation of decision-making authority,

6. financial incentives, and

7. abandonment of patients.

Some of these issues and challenges are discussed elsewhere in this chapter. For example, the next question focuses on safeguarding patients from harm by having an adequate nurse-patient ratio. Challenges regarding financial incentives may involve difficulty in getting approval to perform tests and procedures or doing them purely because they provide income. A mechanism must be available that allows for challenge and reversal of policies that constrain professional judgment or forfeit decision-making authority to third-party payers.

6. What are the ethical implications of staffing decisions?

Nursing administration must balance (1) access to care, (2) standards of care, and (3) allocation of resources in making decisions with financial implications. Nursing administration must balance the needs of patients with available resources in order to provide a reasonable quality of care while meeting their fiduciary responsibility to keep the organization open and functioning at optimal level.

If you believe that the nurse to patient ratio is too low, discuss the situation with the nurse manager. To prepare for your discussion, identify staffing patterns in similar units; use Aiken and colleagues (2002) research data that supports the work of registered nurses, as well as increased recruitment costs to the organization that result from high staff turnover. Nurses must provide evidence of the value of their work; they must show that they are cost effective.

7. If I constantly feel overworked and unable to provide the care I know patients need, can I walk off the unit in protest?

Cost-saving measures and the shortage of nurses has significantly increased the workload of nurses, often to the point of compromising patient health, safety, and rights. Leaving the unit without making reasonable arrangements with an appropriate person to continue nursing care is abandonment of the patient. If you are assigned to work in a situation that is beyond your level of physical or professional competence, there are procedures to follow to object to the assignment. Every organization has a grievance policy and procedure; it is important that you follow that process. Each state has policies regarding abandonment; nurses can be charged with abandonment and unprofessional conduct. While nurses have the right and are responsible to protect their own integrity and safety, they are also responsible for patients. Walking off the unit leaves patients in jeopardy and can result in prosecution.

8. Why can't we just give the patients what they need?

The goals of our healthcare system are in conflict. These goals are

1. provision of the best possible care for all,

2. provision of equal care for all,

3. freedom of choice on part of healthcare providers and consumers, and

4. containment of costs.

Most nurses are taught that we must provide the best care to all patients all of the time; we must meet every possible care need. This perfect care was probably never practical or possible. There just aren't enough resources available as health care is only one of many societal goods.

9. How can we control healthcare costs and still provide equitable access to care?

Some advocate the use of principles to control allocation decisions within institutions. Suggested principles are: (1) improvement of health is the primary goal; (2) patients and HMO members are to be informed about aspects of allocation of healthcare resources; (3) patients and members consent to allocation of resources that will affect them; (4) conflicts of interest of those who make allocation decisions should be minimized (Emanuel, 2000). Adherence to these principles should ease access to care and help control costs. Two difficulties persist: most hospitals do not have a defined membership and health care is but one goal of many (such as education, safety, transportation, defense, housing) that government or society must provide so that there is vigorous competition for resources.

Access to care is based on freedom of choice and financial responsibility. During the past year, health care coverage has become a major contention in labor disputes. Unfortunately, most policy makers are pushing for small reforms that will improve access for some but will reduce access for others. Emanuel and Fuchs (2003) argue for universal healthcare vouchers, a system to establish a fair, functional healthcare system in the United States. This system allows for choice and assigns financial responsibility. Others advocate for one or more of the following: (1) controls and strict budgets, (2) competition, (3) innovations in science and medicine that decrease incidence of major diseases, (4) adoption of healthy lifestyles. It is likely that a number of these and other approaches will be needed to develop an effective, just, and affordable healthcare system. Everyone in a morally responsible country should have access to basic care.

10. What does the principle "justice" mean?

Justice is a principle of bioethics that means giving others what is due to them. Fairness and entitlement are used to explain the idea of justice; equitability and appropriateness of treatment are used to interpret justice in health care. Justice is present whenever persons are due to receive benefits or burdens because of their particular circumstances. Distributive justice is used to allocate resources in health care.

11. How do we decide which patients get scarce treatments?

Rationing scarce resources or microallocation is generally based on (1) utilitarian strategy that emphasizes social efficiency and maximal benefit to patients (the most good for the greatest number), or (2) egalitarian strategy that emphasizes the equal worth of persons and fair opportunity. Information such as constituency, progress of science, and prospect of success must also be considered. Constituency refers to social factors that determine patient boundaries (or market segments) such as veterans, geographic boundaries, ability to pay, or some other nonmedical criteria. Progress of science is research oriented and is concerned with the most efficient use of resources. Prospect of success is important because a scarce medical resource should be given to patients who can reasonably be expected to benefit. These are important ideas, especially in light of studies that have demonstrated prevalent race and gender discrimination in healthcare allocation (Bach et al., 2004; Bloche, 2004; Smedley, Smith, & Nelson, 2003; Steinbrook, 2004).

12. How are equitable financial decisions made in health care?

Allocation of funds is a complex process and begins at the national level with partitioning the comprehensive social budget. Included are education and welfare. Next comes allocation within the health budget that consists of health education, nutrition, and sports as well as health care. Allocation within the healthcare budget includes healthcare facilities, healthcare education, and research. Finally, there is allocation of scarce treatments for patients. In 2002, approximately 14% of the GDP (gross domestic product) or $4,500 per capita was spent on health care in the United States. There are many competing interests coupled with limited resources that make just budgeting difficult at best.

13. How, then, do they budget health care?

First, the kinds of healthcare services needed are identified. Then, who is to receive the services and on what basis and who will deliver the services are delineated. How health care will be funded is established. Finally, who will control how those services will be distributed is decided. Consideration of the principle of justice makes the process complex and difficult because the entire process is very political.

14. Managed care and market forces were supposed to improve access to care and control costs. Why hasn't this happened?

Certain characteristics of the free market work against its effectiveness in resource allocation in health care. These characteristics are:

1. imperfect information,

2. third-party payers,

3. gatekeepers,

4. forced purchase (ill and hurt people often can defer or refuse care only at their own risk),

5. lack of competition, and

6. distorted profit motives.

Also, added layers of administration add to expenditures. There are now 45 million people in the U.S. without access to health care, which is up from 37 million in 1990 (Kaiser Commission, 2004), and shows how difficult resource allocation in health care is.

15. Can rationing be just?

To ration means to supply, apportion, or distribute an allotment. Indeed, we have always rationed health care. The challenge comes in how we ration. There must be equitable distribution of health care based on appropriate principles of ethics such as justice, respect for autonomy, beneficence, and non-maleficence.

16. Do we really have a choice in health care?

Choice in the healthcare market is very much an illusion. Employers choose the insurance program in which employees are enrolled. If the business is very large with many employees, the employees may choose among a limited number of insurance plans. There have been many mergers among managed care organizations so that there are fewer organizations from which to choose. These organizations offer very similar plans. Consumers rarely, if ever, have real choices in health care, unless they pay out of their own pockets.

17. We hear so much about access to care, managed care, and ethics. Are principles really applicable?

We live in a society that is, as all societies are, based on customs, laws, and ethical codes. Morality is social in its origins, sanctions, and functions. Principles of ethics help us sort through ethical problems or dilemmas to find solutions and to develop systems that are congruent with or support society's values and the common good. Principles guide us to become a more just society.

18. Healthcare providers sometimes use deception with third-party payers to ensure that patients receive services they believe are needed. Isn't deception lying and unethical?

There is a conflict between the healthcare provider's role as patient advocate and his/her role within organizations that restrict both provider and patient choices over obtaining financial coverage for procedures. It is hard to say that deception can never be justified. The system should be changed to deal better with third-party restrictions. There are temptations to deceive that threaten the integrity and character of healthcare providers causing moral distress and that also threaten fairness in the system.

RESOURCES

Aiken, L. H., Clarke, S. P., Cheung, R. B., Sloane, D. M., & Silber, J. H. (2003). Educational levels of hospital nurses and surgical patient mortality. *Journal of the American Medical Association, 290*(12), 1617–1623.

Aiken, L. H., Clarke, S. P., Sloane, D. M., Sochalski, J., & Silber, J. H. (2002). Hospital nurse staffing and patient mortality, nurse burnout and job dissatisfaction. *Journal of the American Medical Association, 288*(16), 1987–1993.

Alward, R. R., & Camuñas, C. (1991). *The nurse's guide to marketing.* Albany, NY: Delmar Publishing.

American Nurses Association. (2001). *Code for nurses.* Washington, DC: American Nurses Publishing.

Bach, P. B., Pham, H. H., Schrag, D., Tate, R. C., & Hargraves, J. L. (2004). Primary care physicians who treat Blacks and Whites. *New England Journal of Medicine, 351,* 575–584.

Beauchamp, T. L., & Childress, J. F. (2001). *Principles of biomedical ethics* (5th ed.). New York: Oxford University Press.

Bloche, M. (2004). Health care disparities—Science, politics, and race. *New England Journal of Medicine, 350,* 1568–1570.

Camuñas, C. (1998). Guest editorial: Care, professional integrity, and ethics. *Journal of Nursing Administration, 28*(3), 7–9.

Centers for Medicare & Medicaid Services. (2003). *National health expenditures and projections, 1990–2013.* Baltimore: Author. Retrieved April 16, 2005, from http://www.cms.hhs.gov/statistics/nhe/projections-2003/tl.asp

Davis, A. J., Aroskar, M. A., Liaschenko, J., & Drought, T. S. (1997). *Ethical dilemmas and nursing practice* (4th ed.). Stamford, CT: Appleton & Lange.

Emanuel, E. J. (2000). Justice and managed care: Four principles for the just allocation of health care resources. *Hastings Center Report, 30*(3), 8–16.

Emanuel, E. J., & Fuchs, V. R. (2003, November 18). The universal cure. *The New York Times,* p. A25.

Kaiser Commission. (2004). *The Kaiser Commission on Medicare and the uninsured.* (Fact sheet #1420-06). Washington, DC: Kaiser Family foundation. Retrieved April 21, 2005, from http://www.kff.org

O'Toole, M. T. (Ed.) (2003). *Miller-Keane encyclopedia & dictionary of medicine, nursing, & allied health* (7th ed.). Philadelphia: W. B. Saunders.

Smedley, B. D., Smith, A. Y., & Nelson, A. R. (2003). *Unequal treatment: Confronting racial and ethnic disparities in health care.* Washington, DC: National Academies Press.

Steinbrook, R. (2004). Disparities in health care—From politics to policy. *New England Journal of Medicine, 350,* 1486–1488.

Chapter 18

Organizational Ethics

Mary Lou Helfrich Jones

1. What is the difference between clinical ethics and organizational ethics?

Clinical ethics focuses on an individual patient and addresses the ethical problems that arise in the care of patients. These ethical issues center on end-of-life decisions, withdrawal/withholding of care, cost and allocation of resources, patient rights, quality of life, and futility. A clinical ethical dilemma emerges when there is a conflict between two equally acceptable and competing rights, responsibilities, values, or decisions.

On the other hand, organizational ethics relates to behavioral norms and codes of conduct in institutions. There are some clinical ethics issues that have organizational implications, such as confidentiality, disclosure, truth telling, conflicts of interest, and informed consent. Significant organizational ethics issues are impaired nursing practice, delegation to non-professionals, disruptive physicians, discretion and control, allocation of resources, and human relations.

2. What aspects of the ANA (2001) *Code of Ethics for Nurses With Interpretive Statements* relate to organizational ethics?

All nine provisions of the *Code of Ethics* have implications for clinical and organizational ethics as they make explicit the primary goals, values, and obligations of the profession. As one reflects on each of the nine provisions of the *Code of Ethics*, the statements are prescriptive for nursing, providing a framework for practice. In any practice setting, there is a clinical dimension for actual clinical practice. At the same time, nursing practice is performed within an organizational context.

To illustrate, let's consider two examples. One provision states, "The nurse, in all professional relationships, practices with compassion and respect for the inherent dignity, worth and uniqueness of every individual, unrestricted by considerations of social or economic status, personal attributes or the nature of health problems" (ANA, 2001, p. 7). The interpretive statements illustrate the context of this provision in the relationship with patients and with colleagues in an organization. This perspective is observable in the clinical setting, for example, where the staff nurse serves on a multidisciplinary committee that has weekly patient care planning meetings to manage a high-risk obstetric population. The nurse who knows the patient's complex needs and assertively speaks to these needs in the weekly care plan meetings contributes to this patient's care, supporting safety, and clinical quality. What one sees as an outcome is the collaboration among multiple disciplines to achieve quality health care.

Another perspective with significant organizational ethics implications of the *Code of Ethics* can be found in provision six, which states, "The nurse participates in establishing, maintaining, and improving health care environments and conditions of employment conducive to the provision of quality health care and consistent with the values of the profession through individual and collective action" (ANA, 2001, p. 20). You can see this perspective in action through shared governance-type structures, where the nurse has an active part in developing guidelines on evidence-based care, such as clinical practice councils and performance improvement councils. Other related structures for work environment enhancement include education councils for education program development, scheduling councils for innovative methods to enhance balanced time schedules, and retention councils. Moreover, one sees evidence of this provision in environments where respectful interactions occur on multiple levels, decision making is inclusive related to practice and working conditions, and where patient rights and safe practices are the norm.

3. What standards from the Joint Commission on Accreditation of Healthcare Organizations (JCAHO) are relevant to organizational ethics?

The JCAHO added accreditation standards for organizational ethics in 1995. The areas of focus are related to the formation of a code of ethics for billing, patient transfer, marketing, contractual obligations, and professional relationships within and beyond the healthcare organization. The JCAHO is concerned with the effects of an organization's activities on individual patient care.

The American Hospital Association launched an Organizational Ethics Initiative in 1997 to support healthcare organizations' efforts to make organizational ethics an integral part of the organization through education and consultation. As a result, some Institutional Ethics committees expanded their role to integrate organizational ethics issues to the long-standing clinical ethics issues. Self-education, policy development, and collaborative teams have focused on the organizational ethics of clinical patient care with institution-wide implications. And, a few established Organizational Ethics Committees/Subcommittees. To gain skills in managing organizational ethics issues, these committees undertake self-education along with policy development. For example, to address a specific organizational concern, such as management of charity care, a team of multiple constituencies is formed to process the competing ethical issues and create guidelines to establish and manage such a program. Subsequently, an education and communication plan is designed and implemented.

4. What is an example of organizational ethics?

For example, the charge nurse on an Obstetric Unit is making patient assignments. She has had two nurses call out for the shift and there is no one on call. On evaluation of patient acuity and volume, she determines the need for one more registered nurse. At report, the charge nurse announces the dilemmas of being one RN short and makes an assignment of patients to staff that exceed their capacity. The team assertively confronts the charge nurse requesting additional help. The charge nurse knows she will be reprimanded by the Nurse Manager if she calls for more help. The solution chosen by this charge nurse was to ask one of the staff whose shift is ending to work an additional 4 to 6 hours and to call a staff member on the next shift to come in 4 to 6 hours early. This solution worked. The issue remaining to be resolved is the fear the charge nurse has of a reprimand for ensuring safe staffing.

5. How does an organization support patients and staff when there are conflicts of interest, for example, a patient's refusal to accept blood products?

A nurse is assigned to a pregnant patient who is 30 weeks' gestation with significant anemia. The physician has ordered a blood transfusion, and the patient has declined explaining it is against her religious beliefs. The patient's physician has requested a court order to administer this blood transfusion because of the potential adverse effect on the fetus. The nurse wants to support this patient's wishes and does not want to administer the blood transfusion. She communicates her request to the Charge Nurse to have a different patient assignment. However, it would be important to have communicated her preferences to the Nurse Manager when considering the position during the hiring process.

The fifth provision in the *Code of Ethics* speaks clearly to this situation. When a nurse is placed in a situation of compromise with a particular treatment, intervention, or activity that is morally objectionable, the nurse is justified in refusing to participate. When this situation occurs, the nurse must communicate in appropriate ways. Ideally, these situations should be known in advance, preferably when hired, so appropriate arrangements can be made for patient assignments. When this situation surfaces, it should be clear that alternative plans are implemented. However, the nurse is obligated to provide for the patient's safety, to avoid abandonment, and to withdraw from care only when assured that alternate sourcing of nursing care is available.

6. What is the ethical responsibility of a professional nurse when she observes a co-worker diverting controlled substances? Is it different if it is the Nurse Manager or physician diverting?

When you observe a professional nurse diverting controlled substances, you are obligated by the *Code of Ethics* to express your concern to the nurse you observed. In confronting this nurse, do so privately and state the observations, expressing concern over the possible detrimental/adverse affect on the patient's well-being/safety as well as the integrity of the nurse's practice. You would need to tell this nurse that you must report the incident to the Nurse Manager and encourage the person to join in the interaction with the Nurse Manager. You will also need to be prepared for this nurse to be angry and be able to seek assistance. Finally, support her in getting assistance for her problem through the Employee Assistance Program.

This same confrontation would be expected of a coworker/peer, nurse manager, or a physician. When it is the impaired practice of the nurse manager, contact Human Resources (HR) for guidance. When a physician is involved, you may choose to contact the Nurse Manager so he/she can intervene within the institution's HR policies and guidelines and provide the needed assistance.

7. How does a professional nurse manage a situation when a colleague/peer delivers patient care that is contradictory to standard of practice?

A professional nurse should address a coworker when he/she observes a practice that is contradictory to the standard of nursing practice. If an intervention can occur prior to actually carrying out the practice, that would be preferable. Confronting a colleague is best done privately. However, in an emergent, life-threatening situation, you may be in a situation where privacy is not an option. In that set of circumstances, asking the nurse to stop what he/she is about to do may be your only recourse. A respectful approach is desirable, but you must be firm and insistent to promote patient safety.

Following the emergent situation, a discussion with the nurse and the immediate supervisor will be important to address performance and provide remediation as needed and appropriate.

8. How does a professional nurse manage a patient care situation when a peer has given direction to a non-professional team member that should not be performed by a non-professional person?

I would approach the nurse with the intent to gain understanding of the rationale for this direction/delegation. By doing this, I would be able to provide coaching, education, and respectful guidance for future situations. If this can be done successfully, then one achieves a positive outcome for team building. Additionally, reporting such an occurrence to the immediate supervisor is important, particularly if you meet any resistance or the incident has occurred before. This action will help the individual understand the seriousness of the situation and gain education and coaching. This situation is referenced in the ANA (2001) *Code of Ethics* perspective that states, "The nurse is responsible and accountable for individual nursing practice and determines the appropriate delegation of tasks consistent with the nurse obligations to provide optimum patient care" (ANA, 2001, p. 16).

9. What is the ethical responsibility of a staff nurse when he/she is confronted by an angry physician who is verbally abusive?

As part of my orientation to the institution, I would have learned the appropriate steps to take in confronting a verbally abusive physician and reporting such behavior. It is a challenge to do so; yet I would walk away from the physician, telling him/her that I would not listen, particularly in a patient's presence. I would reference the administrative policy guiding appropriate steps with a disruptive practitioner, such as contacting the charge nurse, nurse manager on the shift, or contacting the supervisor on duty for the shift.

I would speak with this physician in a private place if I felt safe to do so. If I didn't feel safe, I would contact my immediate supervisor first to participate in a discussion with this physician. In that discussion, I would describe the behavior and the impact on me, so the physician would understand.

If I am the person in charge in a clinical area, I would contact the next level of administrative personnel. I would follow up and document the interaction, on the appropriate form, using factual, objective statements.

10.   How does a nurse respond to a physician who approached him/her to be involved with a medical device company who wants to bring the device in on a weekend to "try out" during a patient procedure?

I would use my knowledge of the institutional policies and procedures that provide clear direction when a request such as this is made. Such a policy is usually found in the administrative policy and procedure manual. Usually the physician is referred to the Institutional Review Board (IRB) or Department Chairperson. These guidelines may include what to say, who to refer the physician to, and support/encouragement to do this. If written guidelines are not immediately available, then I would contact my immediate supervisor to seek assistance and guidance, using the IRB guidelines and administrative policies and procedures.

11.   What does a staff nurse do when a pharmaceutical representative contacts her/him and asks for time at a staff meeting to promote/display that company's products and offers a gratuity of a clinical conference (registration, travel, and hotel expenses)?

I would respond to this request by declining to participate in this effort, based on the institution's policy regarding procedures for any medical company representative to make contact with institutional staff. In most organizations, there is a clear policy regarding the process for a pharmaceutical representative to enter an institution and with whom the representative may interact. The entry point is usually a Purchasing/Procurement Department where the person's credentials are validated and authorization to enter is provided based on verification of appointments with relevant departments. The offering of a gratuity to gain access to a group of staff to promote a product in a staff meeting is a conflict of interest and is unethical/unacceptable behavior.

12. What does a professional nurse do when he/she observes a colleague/peer performing care that violates standards of clinical practice?

It is crucial for a professional nurse, as a member of the clinical team, to be assertive, respectful, and directly inform the team member when a sterile, surgical technique has been broken, or any other procedure is performed in violation of a standard whether a colleague, peer, nurse manager, or physician. The positive atmosphere to promote this timely communication is essential. If negative consequences occur when these situations are confronted, then the nurse should seek the supervisor's support. If the support doesn't exist, then the nurse would appropriately question whether he/she is practicing in a desirable, ethical environment. In such a situation, seeking assistance and coaching from a trusted colleague or professional association may be helpful in reaching an acceptable solution.

13. What should a professional nurse's approach be if there is a conflict regarding a patient care assignment with the immediate supervisor?

I would suggest you discuss this conflict with the immediate supervisor, ask what his/her concern is, and then explain the disagreement with the assignment. It will be important to ensure that the patient will not be in jeopardy, should you not take the patient assignment, as this would constitute abandonment and is a violation of most states' nurse practice acts and the ANA (2001) *Code of Ethics for Nurses*.

14. How does a professional nurse get involved in creating a positive ethical climate?

As a professional nurse, I have the responsibility and accountability to demonstrate behaviors that display the norms of professionalism, trust, integrity, respect for the inherent dignity, worth, and uniqueness of every individual, and all associated behaviors articulated in the ANA (2001) *Code of Ethics for Nurses*. These behaviors, along with a commitment to demonstrate clinical and operational competencies in nursing practice are critical to support a positive ethical climate where staff members are supported and can grow professionally. Offer to serve as a member of the Ethics Committee or a committee that supports ethics like the personnel committee or shared governance committees.

15. How can I report unethical situations if I want to remain unidentified, for fear of losing my job?

In healthcare organizations today, there are compliance departments, sometimes labeled integrity programs. In these departments and programs, there are guidelines provided for individuals to anonymously report situations that may be unethical, and potentially illegal. Sometimes there are hotlines where a person can leave a message. There are also ways to submit written documents of concern. Appropriate care to report the situation accurately and factually is essential. In these compliance programs, there are consequences for reporting information that is untruthful or not accurate because of the significant impact a report can have.

16. What is my ethical responsibility when I think Medicare coding fraud is occurring? Do I have whistleblower's protection?

It is essential that organizations comply with coding and billing practices under the laws that govern Federal and state-funded healthcare programs, and with the requirements of third-party payers. If I think that Medicare coding fraud is occurring, then I would report this to the immediate supervisor, or report to the compliance office in the organization, anonymously or directly. In most organizations today, with the requirement to have compliance offices, whistleblower protection exists (as part of the regulations).

17. Case: I know two of my colleagues are repeatedly calling in sick because they are tired from a second job. The nurse manager does not know and is being severely criticized for not managing overtime expenses. What is my ethical responsibility?

I would follow the policies of the organization regarding reporting of such behavior, an ethical obligation to tell the truth and protect the patients affected. Knowing these two nurses are repeatedly calling in sick generates a concern for the patients on the unit. And, I would be assertive and speak to my colleagues, especially since the nurse manager is not aware. Additionally, I would report these occurrences to the nurse manager.

18. What if I report an ethics problem but the supervisor does nothing?

If the supervisor does nothing when I have reported an ethics problem, I can follow a chain of communication to the next levels of supervision outlined in the institution's established processes (e.g., Department Head, Divisional Director, Chief Operations Officer, and Chief Executive Officer). If the organization has a hotline for reporting problems and I am uncomfortable reporting overtly to meet my legal responsibility, then I can use the hotline. It is important to note that fear of reprisal does not remove the obligation to report any threats to patient safety. I can also contact the local or state professional nursing organization/association to seek guidance, as well, on the appropriate steps to take.

19. What is the ethical responsibility of a nurse when observing a colleague access records on a patient he/she is not caring for?

This access is illegal and violates the Health Information Portability Accessibility and Accountability Act (HIPPA). As a nurse, I would confront my colleague, physician, or supervisor and inform them that accessing records on a patient not under their care is not permissible and is a Federal violation of patient privacy and confidentiality. Institutions have adopted disciplinary procedures when such as action occurs. I would be obligated to inform them that I must report this activity.

RESOURCES

American Nurses Association. (2001). *Code of ethics for nurses with interpretive statements*. Washington, DC: American Nurses Publishing.

Bales, M. D. (1989). *Professional ethics* (2nd ed.). Belmont, CA: Wadsworth Publishing Company.

Boyles, P. K., DuBose, E. R., Ellingson, S. J., Guinn, D. E., & McCurdy, D. B. (2001). *Organizational ethics in health care: Principles, cases, and practical solutions.* San Francisco, CA: Jossey-Bass Publishers.

Browner, M. M., & Keeley, S. M. (1994). *Asking the right questions: A guide to critical thinking.* Englewood Cliffs, NJ: Prentice-Hall.

Coughlin, S. S., Soskolne, C. L., & Goodman, K. W. (1997). *Case studies in public health ethics.* Washington, DC: American Public Health Association.

Ethics Resource Center. Organizational Ethics Page. www.ethics.org/business ethics.html

Ketefian, S. (1988). *Moral reasoning and ethical practice in nursing: An integrative review.* New York: National League for Nursing.

Mills, A. E., Spencer, E. M., & Werhane, P. H. (Eds.). (2001). *Developing organization ethics in healthcare: A case-based approach to policy, practice and compliance.* Hagerstown, MD: University Publishing Group, Inc.

Park Ridge Center Bulletin. (1998). Special issue on Organizational Ethics. Issue 3, February/March. www.parkridgecenter.org/Page554.html

Spencer, E. M., Mills, A. E., Rorty, M. V., & Werhane, P. H. (2000). *Organization ethics in health care.* New York: Oxford University Press.

Sugerman, J. (2000). *Ethics in primary care.* New York: McGraw-Hill.

Chapter 19

Leadership Ethics

Kathy Malloch

1. How does a leader determine when a decision is ethically congruent with the provision of healthcare services?

Nurse leaders are continually faced with multiple priorities and multiple options in which the "right" approach is seldom evident. Nurse leaders can enhance their decision-making skills with careful consideration to the patient's needs as the primary focus, assurance of patient care services that are therapeutic, and avoiding decisions that may benefit the organization at the expense of patient comfort, safety, and quality. This is not to imply that the nurse leader should not be fiscally responsible, but rather that the nurse leader's role is to first create value for the patient and second to assure that those services are within the resources of the organization. Necessarily, when there is a gap between the needed patient services and available fiscal and staff resources, the role of the nurse leader is to create new dialogue with other leaders to address the gap.

2. *Case:* Nurses on the unit are very concerned about bio-terrorism readiness, specifically what to do about smallpox vaccination for themselves. The nurse manager informed the nurses that bio-terrorism in this service is not a priority at this time and there really isn't anything to worry about. How should nurses address this situation?

Oftentimes when the workload of the nurse manager is high, one more task added to the pile is overwhelming. Employees have the right to receive relevant information. Given that the information is essential for nurses in their caregiver roles and as patient educators, the nurse manager is accountable to address this concern. To facilitate the process, staff nurses should create a list of their questions about smallpox vaccination for the nurse manager and then ask for assistance. Another option is to identify a reference source—book, video, or speaker—that could present the information to the nurses and request that the nurse manager arrange to obtain the information.

3. *Case:* **The organization discourages nurses from becoming members of the American Nurses Association (ANA) because of its commitment to collective bargaining. Nurses want to join as they believe the Association sets the standards for nursing practice and believe their participation on ANA committees is a professional obligation. How should this be addressed?**

Nurses are hired by organizations on the basis of their nursing skill and knowledge that is based on the American Nurses Association standards and principles. Participation in and commitment to professional standards and principles is an essential characteristic of the nurse. While the bargaining arm of ANA is problematic to many human resource directors, it is important to note that the ANA also has a commitment to workplace advocacy in the professional arm of the organization. Each nurse should work to educate those in the organization who resist professional membership with information that clearly describes the essence of the ANA. Failure to resolve this issue may require the nurse to seek a more supportive employer.

4. Is having all decisions related to patient care practices approved by the chief financial officer appropriate?

The role of the financial officer has emerged from a staff support role to an operational decision-making role over the past 20 years, most likely a result of decreasing reimbursement and increasing competition. All operational and line positions require knowledge skills and abilities that support the provision of health care. Operational positions are held by healthcare employees accountable for ensuring that service, quality, and outcomes are present. A staff position, such as the chief financial officer position, should *support* the work of operations, rather than direct the work. Performing both roles assumes knowledge and experience in both the clinical and financial areas.

Ideally, decisions specific to the use of resources should be made on the basis of value to patient outcomes. The question should be, *does the expenditure or lack of expenditure improve or contribute to the desired patient care outcomes?* Clinical evidence is required from caregivers to support such decisions. Unfortunately, evidence for practice and outcomes is just beginning to emerge in the literature (Aiken et al., 1994; Aiken et al., 2002; Buerhaus & Needleman, 2000). The appropriate strategy is for the team of caregivers, managers, and financial officers to make decisions collaboratively on what is the best balance to achieve patient quality and work within available resources.

5. Are sign-on bonuses appropriate? If dollars are available, shouldn't they be spent on existing employees, not potential employees?

Oftentimes in desperation, organizations use economic enticements to recruit needed healthcare workers. The *bonus model* for employees is an unfortunate devaluing of healthcare professionals to a level that portrays them as shallow and materialistic individuals. Some individuals will respond to the enticement of the financial bonus in given situations, but the reality is that most healthcare professionals are motivated by a combination of social, emotional, and material needs and are not led by the dollar. Sign-on bonuses are a recruitment tool for an individual of unknown performance. Focusing on retention of current employees who are known entities is a more appropriate use of scarce dollars. Creating a culture of shared leadership, respect, and fair compensation far exceeds the value of a sign-on bonus.

6. *Case:* The chief nursing officer (CNO) has supported the implementation of a shared governance council structure and informed nurses that their decision making and processes will be respected. Nurses have become concerned because the CNO has begun to override policy decisions and change priorities of the council. What should nurses do about this situation?

The adage of *walking the talk* in this situation can be the ultimate challenge for the leaders schooled in command and control behaviors. Learning to transition to the role of coach, mentor, and guide is difficult for even the most committed leader. The appropriate approach is a direct one since discussing the problem without the CNO would be counterproductive. Pointing out the observed behavior to the CNO and asking for guidance on how to manage the situation is the first step. Assuming that the CNO is unaware of the behavior and given his/her commitment to a shared leadership model, this discussion will result in increased awareness and a change in behavior. If the CNO rationalizes that this approach is necessary, further discussion is warranted to determine what shared leadership means to the CNO and how such situations should be managed.

7. *Case:* **Nurse managers are required to attend the safety committee on a monthly basis, even though they do not believe their opinions are valued or considered in forming policies. The CEO says all meetings are needed; yet the team believes that is not true. What are the responsibilities of the team?**

    The author Steve Kaye noted that businesses waste an average of 20% of their professional payroll on bad meetings (1998). Meetings that consist of only one-way communication or information giving should be eliminated in favor of memos or e-mail. Face-to-face meetings should be held when there is a need for dialogue and problem solving.
      The team should review its goals, purposes, and expected outcomes and determine the most appropriate method to get the intended work completed. With this information, the team can determine if a face-to-face meeting or electronic communication or a combination are the most useful. Each team member then assumes accountability for reviewing electronic communications in a timely manner and responding as needed. In addition, electronic communication should never replace situations in which healthy dialogue is needed. Each method, electronic and face-to-face communication, has advantages and disadvantages.

8. *Case:* **Nurse managers have been competing with each other for highest patient satisfaction scores— those with lower but satisfactory scores are being**

identified as low performers. What's wrong with this approach?

Competing between patient care units necessarily results in one winner and the others losers—an adversarial environment at best. Patient satisfaction varies among patient populations; post-partum, medical surgical units, and ambulatory care each have distinct benchmarks and needs. Attempting to compare the satisfaction scores on a post-partum unit with those of a medical unit is inappropriate. The more appropriate approach is to use an internal benchmarking approach; the post-partum unit should set performance targets and continually work to exceed those targets. The medical unit should do likewise.

9. *Case:* The leader works to shield employees from unpleasant news about finance, adverse outcomes, and quality performance scores, leaving employees to learn about negative information in the newspaper or from colleagues in other healthcare facilities. Why should employees hear organizational news first?

Too often information that is believed confidential "leaks" out to the public resulting in perceptions of dishonesty, lack of timely information sharing, and avoidance of conflict. Employees have the right to be free to say what is needed to be said about an issue and to be free to disagree with one another in order to increase their understanding of issues. Hearing bad news is never pleasant, but it is worse when individuals are left in the dark to assume something even worse than the bad news. Selective sharing of information negatively affects effective, trusting working relationships. Building trusting relationships among employees requires openness and sharing of both positive and negative information. Trusting relationships ultimately improve organizational performance.

10. *Case:* The manager is very concerned about overtime and has instructed nurses to clock out at the end of the shift. If there is more work (charting) to be done, the nurse is told to work on personal organization and priority setting skills and complete the

charting "off the clock." Is this an acceptable practice?

The pressure to meet budget targets should never override acceptable practices. The practice described is not acceptable for two reasons. First, it is inconsistent with Federal labor laws and second, failing to understand and manage the workload reflects a serious leadership need. This practice reflects the larger, unresolved, and ever-present problem of too much work and too little time. The manager is challenged to evaluate the work that is being done to ensure that it is appropriate and positively influences patient outcomes. New strategies to manage the variance between the required work and available staff need to be created by the healthcare team, not the individual nurse at the bedside.

11. *Case:* **The manager consistently decreases daily staffing in order to meet budget guidelines. Errors are increasing and patient care is negatively affected. Should I report the manager to the state board of nursing for failure to delegate, supervise, and protect patient safety?**

The first approach should be to state the problem as clearly as possible to the manager. If that does not yield results and patient care continues to be negatively affected, the nurse is obligated to go up the chain of command to communicate the concerns and the evidence of poor patient outcomes. The chain of command includes the charge nurse, supervisor, unit director, division director, chief nursing officer, and chief executive officer of the organization. If these efforts do not yield changes that affect patient care positively, the nurse may choose to report the situation to the board of nursing on the belief that the nurse manager and others have failed to protect patient safety through the appropriate delegation and supervision of work processes.

12. *Case:* **Most nurses on the unit refuse to precept new nurses because they don't have enough time and also believe that nurses should be better prepared by the schools before coming to work. What should be done about this situation?**

A group approach to this situation is recommended. First, determine what it would take to have nurses mentor new nurses. This approach is different from asking the question, "Why don't nurses want to mentor new nurses?" Determining the obstacles and strategies can reverse the negative processes. Second, a review of the American Nurses Association (2001) *Code of Ethics* can be helpful. The *Code* serves as a reminder of the commitment of each nurse to the profession and the development of novice nurses.

Socialization to the unit and orientation to practice are equally important in retaining nurses. A nurse with good technical skills is unlikely to remain with an employer if there is an attitude of "figure it out for yourself."

Finally, feedback specific to the preparation of nurses should be given by the organization to the college(s) of nursing. Faculty and managers should hold regular meetings to review concerns and work collaboratively to resolve the deficiency.

13. *Case:* **The nurse leader is Hispanic and shows favoritism toward other Hispanic nurses. She believes that if she doesn't give the nurses the schedule days they want they will quit and there will be less diversity in the team. What is wrong with this strategy?**

    Equitable practices that support the work and mission of the organization should be the goal of leaders. The ethical condition of inclusion is met when those who have a stake in the outcome of a decision are included in the decision-making process. Given that all nurses have a stake in the scheduling process, the exclusion of selected (non-Hispanic) nurses will most likely result in an imbalance in scheduling and overall staff dissatisfaction. Attempting to meet the needs of one group over the needs of another is shortsighted and will have negative long-term effects. An open discussion with all team members to determine the fairest approach is the appropriate strategy. Behind the scenes negotiating and deal making destroys trust.

14. *Case:* **An experienced staff nurse is uncomfortable delegating tasks to a specific LP/VN because he believes the nurse does not practice safely, so he does the work himself, which results in his being overwhelmed. Why is this approach unethical?**

    This approach is unethical because it is a misuse of organizational resources and demonstrates a lack of accountability to supervision, as articulated as necessary in the ANA (2001) *Code of Ethics*. Practice based on evidence rather than personal preferences is always desirable. When there is reluctance to delegate, the root cause is more often lack of knowledge of delegation-supervision principles and accountability. Lack of patience is simply a symptom of the lack of knowledge, not the root cause. Basic delegation skills include knowing the state nurse practice act, assessment of the situation, planning for the delegation, ensuring appropriate accountability, supervising performance of the task, and evaluation of the delegation process. Too often nurses fail to intervene when task performance is unsatisfactory through communication with the leaders/managers of the unit. The result is that nurses minimize appropriate delegation and take on overwhelming workloads that are nearly impossible to complete.

15. *Case:* **The oncology unit always gets new equipment and better staffing because the oncology physicians complain more than other physicians. What should happen in this situation? What should the nurse do?**

Once again, open discussion that focuses on the organization's mission and goals rather than on selected needs requires inclusion of those with a stake in the outcome of decisions. In this case, the allocation of funding for new equipment is an issue for many stakeholders; thus, their inclusion in the discussion and decision-making process is the right thing to do.

Further, the imbalance of power between stakeholders in this situation cannot be ignored. Strong-willed stakeholders may assert their power; however, failure to channel this power into a group decision-making process will lead to disenfranchisement and loss of organizational energy and synergy. Pulling together the nurses who are interested in this issue, determining ways to collect the facts on the issue, and finally planning a strategy are all necessary beginning steps.

16. *Case:* **An experienced nurse administered an overdose of medication that resulted in serious patient instability and the need for additional therapeutic interventions. The nurse was suspended and eventually terminated for unsafe practice based upon hospital policy. Is this policy or practice acceptable in**

health care? Given the situation above should the nurse or nurse manager inform the patient of the error?

No nurse ever enters the profession of nursing to harm a patient. Given the inevitability of error in a human system, reacting to mistakes punitively is unlikely to minimize their occurrence, even though our culture leads us to expect the assignment of blame, correction of the error, and in most cases, punishment of those who make the mistake. Attaching blame to individuals creates a climate of shame and guilt and further decreases candid reporting and discussion of mistakes.

Punishment of error makers fails to produce the desired results, namely, the elimination of error. The emphasis should be on recognizing and recovering from the error to learn from mistakes, to identify actions that will decrease the chance of repeating the same mistakes, and to improve performance as well. The goal should always be to strive for excellence, not the unrealistic expectation of perfection given the uncontrollable variables present in the healthcare system.

Disclosure of errors is embedded in the ethics manual of the American College of Physicians (Snyder & Leffler, 2005). The manual notes that errors do not necessarily constitute improper, negligent, or unethical behavior, but failure to disclose them may. The disclosure of errors provides the opportunity to recognize "brokenness." While acknowledging errors may be morally required, the current litigious culture makes it nearly impossible for care providers to willingly divulge mistakes. The culture is moving toward disclosure and greater accountability; however, the nurse should discuss the process of disclosure with the administrative team prior to discussing the error with a patient or the family.

17. *Case:* **Staffing shortages and the lack of available registered nurses have resulted in very stressful and unsafe conditions. The nurse manager makes rounds on all shifts and helps with the workload whenever possible imploring nurses to "do their best." Why is this an inappropriate strategy?**

Once again, the challenge is to manage reality—the reality that there are not always enough staff to complete the work in the allotted time frame. Even the most valid and reliable patient classification system and scheduling practices cannot assure that the right number of nurses will be available at the right time. New systems and expectations are required to manage this inevitable situation without abandoning the individual nurse to do his/her best.

Attempting to provide all services regardless of the available resources, as has been the practice, is irresponsible. Selected strategies need to be created by the team. These include:

1. ensure that the staffing system is indeed valid and reliable,

2. eliminate non-value added services,

3. delay non-critical functions until staff are available,

4. decrease the frequency of monitoring of stable patients, and

5. re-route any new admissions to other areas.

18. Peer review is a process used for evaluations. Three colleagues provide input, but policy does not allow the nurse to know specific feedback from each individual providing input. Is it unfair to withhold such information?

Open, honest dialogue about performance leads to better performance. Withholding or masking feedback behind an average rating within a 360-degree evaluation process decreases an individual's opportunity to modify behaviors and reinforces the standard that open, direct communication is not an expectation. This policy should be modified to require open, honest sharing of feedback. Holding back information is an oppressive leadership behavior and prevents others from managing their own behavior.

RESOURCES

Aiken, L. H., Clark, S. P., Sloane, D. M., Sochalski, J., & Silber, J. H. (2002). Hospital nurse staffing and patient mortality, nurse burnout, and job dissatisfaction. *Journal of the American Medical Association, 288*(16), 1987–1993.

Aiken, L. H., Smith, H. L., & Lake, E. T. (1994). Lower Medicare mortality among a set of hospitals known for good nursing care. *Medical Care, 32*(8), 771–787.

American Organization of Nurse Executives. www.aone.org

Bagley, C. E. (2002). The ethical leader's decision tree. *Harvard Business Review*, *80*(2), 18–20.

Buerhaus, P., & Needleman, J. (2000). Policy implication of research on nurse staffing and quality of care. *Policy, Politics & Nursing Practice*, *1*(1), 5–16.

Cooper, R. W., Frank, G. L., Gouty, C. A., & Hanen, M. C. (2002). Key ethical issues encountered in healthcare organizations. *Journal of Nursing Administration*, *32*(6), 331–337.

Kaye, S. (1998). Effective meetings: A whole brain approach. Retrieved January 30, 2004. http://www.stevekaye.com/facilitator.htm

Melnyk, B. M., & Fineout-Overholt, E. (2005). *Evidence based practice in nursing and healthcare: A guide to best practice*. Philadelphia: Lippincott, Williams & Wilkins.

National Center for Health Care Leadership. www.nchl.org

Porter-O'Grady, T., & Malloch, K. (2002). *Quantum leadership: A textbook of new leadership*. Sudbury, MA: Jones & Bartlett Publishers.

Reiser, S. J. (1994). The ethical life of health care organizations. *The Hastings Center Report*, *24*(6), 28–35.

Snyder, L., & Leffler, C. (2005). Ethics manual (5th ed.). *Annals of Internal Medicine*, *142*, 560–582. http://www.acponline.org/ethics/ethicsman.htm

Chapter 20

Labor Ethics

Vicki D. Lachman and Julia W. Aucoin

1. What is the focus of labor ethics?

Work environments provide numerous opportunities for conflicts between management and staff rights. Personnel policies, job descriptions, and even union contracts are designed to clarify responsibilities. However, ethical resolution of issues requires a process where all can be heard, a value of fairness, and a continuous search for equitable solutions. Enron and Allegany Healthcare are examples of not only corruption at the top, but a lack of ethical management of labor. Examples of labor ethics issues include e-mail monitoring, how employees with chronic diseases are supported, and how short staffing is fixed.

2. *Case:* Since 9/11, my organization has really been monitoring our e-mail system to the point where I feel like my privacy is being invaded. What are my rights to privacy? If they are being violated, what are my options?

Prior to 9/11 the basic Federal protection for privacy of electronic communications was found in the Electronic Communication Privacy Act (ECPA) of 1986. With the passage of the USA Patriotic Act, 2001, Federal legislation was designed to enhance national security and expanded electronic workplace monitoring of e-mail, computer files, Internet activity, and telephone calls. Software can reveal the online activities of employees, including Web sites visited and length of employees' visits to Web sites. Software may also be used to monitor employees' computer hard-drive to identify pornography, music, or movies that have been downloaded in violation of copyright laws or workplace policy. U.S. workers are not generally protected from surveillance on the grounds that the premises and equipment are possessions of the employer and the employee can have no legitimate expectations of privacy.

3. **Case: I have one of the unseen chronic illnesses— multiple sclerosis. Some days I am so fatigued that I have a hard time keeping up the pace. The hospital has a right to expect me to perform as everyone else, doesn't it?**

Multiple sclerosis is similar to other diseases such as chronic fatigue syndrome, endometriosis, fibromyalgia, HIV, colitis, Crohn's disease, irritable bowel syndrome, migraine headaches, asthma, arthritis, epilepsy, depression, schizophrenia, or nephritis. This list is not intended to be comprehensive, but suggests the number and variability of conditions which may be described as unseen.

People with chronic conditions may be placed in situations of "role insufficiency" where they fear being unable to meet the perceived role obligations. Role models for aspiring careerists can be portrayed as high-energy, high-performance individuals who are unconstrained by anything, particularly illness and disability. There is a lack of role expectations for the chronically ill, especially for people with unseen chronic illness who may not wish to disclose their condition.

However, in most organizations there is an unwritten rule, as well as the Americans With Disabilities Act that expects organizations to provide "reasonable accommodations." Too often, it is the individual who is unwilling to ask colleagues for assistance when he/she needs it and blames him/herself for not doing enough. The desire to look normal is often overshadowed by the existence of real illness limitations. I would suggest that you learn who would support you and who you could reasonably ask for help. You are most likely to find humanitarian concern from your colleagues. More recent emphasis on organizational ethics and morality are also likely to help you receive other's beneficence.

4. *Case:* I work the night shift in Critical Care and have recently been doing a lot of extra shifts because of an extreme shortage of RNs. I am now sleep deprived because I have worked five 12-hour shifts in a row. Doesn't the organization bear some responsibility if I make a mistake?

The National Commission on Sleep Disorders research reports that sleep loss impairs performance on cognitive tasks involving memory, learning, logical reasoning, arithmetic calculations, pattern recognition, complex verbal processing, and decision making (Oexman, Knotts, & Koch, 2002). For example, reduction of sleep time to 5 hours a night for only 2 nights significantly reduces physiological levels of alertness, impairs vigilance, and worsens arithmetic ability and creative thinking. A loss of as little as 3 hours of sleep in a single night can slow human reaction time significantly, a change that can be dangerous in the stressful conditions of a Critical Care Unit. Research indicates a coping problem could occur with more than five shifts in a row without off-time, 12-hour shifts involving critical monitoring tasks, and more than four 12-hour night shifts in a row. Given your schedule, you can see that you are vulnerable to making a mistake.

The organization could also bear some responsibility under the legal term *respondeat superior.* This doctrine of law holds the employer responsible for the legal consequences of the acts of employees while the employee acts within the scope of employment. However, if you make a mistake that ends in a malpractice case, then you will also be held liable.

5. *Case:* The hospital has nurses participate in decision making, but I do not see employment conditions improving. Now I am expected to share my knowledge as a preceptor, but again without significant rewards. What is management's responsibility, if we are expected to participate to this degree?

Researchers in best practices in the United States found that successful companies were characterized by significant levels of participation by employees on a wide range of matters (Jones, 2002). However, many companies ignore the relationship between employees' rights to improve employment conditions, employee responsibilities in company decision making, and employees' willingness to share knowledge. Despite the rhetoric, there is little evidence of any major long-term increase in employee participation in company decision making. Unless employees are provided with a real opportunity for participation in decision making that improves employees' conditions of employment, they will have little incentive to share their knowledge and assist the organization to become an "intelligent organization."

Hospitals that have reached Magnet status often have shared governance structure in place, which truly facilitates employee participation. In shared governance, employees have an opportunity to make a recommendation, but also the opportunity to be accountable for taking the idea to fruition. In Magnet hospitals most of the rewards are improvements in employee conditions, rather than significant financial personal rewards. However, most organizations increase hourly pay and decrease the nurse-patient ratio for nurses who act as preceptors.

6. The neutral reference policy seems detrimental to former good employees and to the organization, because they end up hiring bad employees. How does an organization ethically justify this stance?

The neutral reference policy (a neutral reference gives the requesting party no information, either positive or negative) has been employers' response to the increasing number of reference defamation suits that have been filed against them by former employees. In fact, a plaintiff who files a reference defamation action against a former employer prevails in 10% of the cases or less. More alarmingly, a neutral response to a reference request is often interpreted as a negative appraisal by prospective employers.

The employer can minimize the risk of reference defamation litigation by documenting the disciplinary actions against and the negative statements about the former employee. Truthful adverse information, carefully investigated and well documented, will not result in liability to a former employer. It is only defamation if the statement that is harmful to the person's reputation is false.

Studies have shown that past job performance is the most accurate measure of future job performance; therefore, a neutral reference policy makes the evaluation of prospective employees extremely difficult. The existence of a duty to report is clear in some situations (e.g., embezzlement, sexual harassment, drug abuse) than in others (e.g., absenteeism, poor work quality, incompetence, poor attitude toward work, chronic tardiness, alcoholism). In summary, the employer's moral duty to disclose is determined by the nature of the employee information being requested by the prospective employer. If, in fact, the employer is "passing along" an employee whose moral fiber is of question, then the neutral reference is unethical.

7. As a healthcare employee, am I protected if I report fraud and negligence?

Whistleblowing involves present or former employees reporting illegal, unethical activities, under the control of organization leaders, to parties who are willing and able to take action to correct the wrongdoing. It is the current position of most managers to recognize that whistleblowers help organizations correct unsafe products/services and working conditions; they also help curb fraudulent practices, and in so doing avoid costly lawsuits and negative publicity for the organization.

An individual's perception of the organization's degree of encouragement of whistleblowing is dependent on the following:

1. knowing where to report fraudulent activities

2. perceiving that the individual will receive a degree of protection from retaliation and reprisal

3. experiencing a supportive climate, where there is a lack of need to control and use status to control situations

Research also supports that individuals with higher levels of moral reasoning are more likely to place themselves in the position of a whistleblower, especially on serious issues such as stealing organizational funds, accepting bribes or kickbacks, or health and safety violations (Keenan, 2002). If your organization meets the criteria listed above, then you are more likely to be protected if you report your concerns. Many organizations have hotlines where issues of corporate compliance are to be reported.

8. *Case:* **We have an Employee Assistance Program (EAP) to help us with difficulties in our lives that affect our work. However, management can force us to go and they get a report of our progress. Does this not break the rules of confidentiality?**

Research supports that in order for an organization to have a successful EAP, management must do the following:

1. express support for the program at various levels

2. purposely educate employees about the program

3. provide necessary training on its use

4. make the program adequately accessible to employees

5. ensure that it operates in a confidential, credible, and neutral manner

6. demonstrate neutrality of the program in organizational politics, especially in labor disputes (Milne, Blum, & Roman, 1994)

Without these characteristics, employees do not have confidence in the EAP. Research repeatedly supports a positive and robust relationship between employee trust and confidence in the EAP and actual use.

It is normal for managers to get reports on compliance, attendance, and follow-through; however, it is highly unusual for a manager to receive any reports on the nature of the problem or progress in the sessions.

9. *Case:* **One of my colleagues just got called into the manager's office because of her "lifestyle off duty" which includes dancing at a bar. Why does management have a right to discipline her for what she does on her own time?**

What you do on your own time is your own business. However, you are a representative of the organization whether you are on the clock or not. While the employer cannot restrict your off-duty lifestyle, it can certainly offer an opinion about it and how it affects the organization negatively. If the activities carry over into the main employment setting (e.g., hangover, positive drug test, or soliciting for the bar), then the employer does have a right to discipline using the progressive discipline plan of the organization. The manager may not know the details of the off-duty lifestyle, but could take the opportunity to clarify any rumors that the manager has heard in this discussion. For example, the employee may be a fully clothed dancer in an adult club or just dancing with someone for relaxation or enjoyment. Only activities that could be harmful to the organization's image or business need be addressed.

10. *Case:* **One of my colleagues has an ill mother and she just adopted a little girl. She is gone more than she is here and we have to accommodate her absences. This does not seem fair, but what can we do?**

According to Federal law, she is allowed leave under the Family Medical Leave Act, 1996 (FMLA). The adoption and the illness are treated as two separate, covered situations. Had they not occurred simultaneously, then there would be little question about the validity of each claim. She is allowed up to 12 weeks for each situation under this Act. While it may not seem fair, it is completely legal and it is her right to use the leave.

In many cases, FMLA abuse is suspected when in fact co-workers may not know all the details of the person's situation. While it seems that co-workers are frustrated about this situation, when placed in a similar position, everyone would want the opportunity to return to the job when this situation was resolved. Obviously, the fact that you are compensated with overtime pay to cover this staffing vacancy is not sufficient. If other of your colleagues are feeling the same way, then it is time to sit down with the nurse manager to discuss other options.

11. *Case:* **I have never been pro-union, but most of my colleagues are seriously considering supporting a union that has approached our organization. I understand why management cannot give us raises and needs to increase our co-pays for health insurance. What can I do to help my colleagues understand the "state of health care"?**

Just because a union approaches the organization doesn't mean that you'll get a raise or a decrease in health insurance co-pay. With a union comes the added expense of union dues and other union obligations. The American Nurses Association has two avenues for supporting staff: The United American Nurses, the only professional nursing union, and the Center for American Nurses, a workplace advocacy organization. Rather than work with a non-nursing union that approaches the organization, it is recommended that you seek assistance from either of these nursing associations as they are familiar with the state of health care and are in the best position to provide guidance. Spending time with colleagues during work and breaks to discuss what you know to be true at other healthcare organizations may provide a much needed perspective on their apparent frustrations.

12. *Case:* **My manager is unfair in how she disciplines staff. She has her favorites and they are untouchable. What recourse do I have to create a fair evaluation climate?**

If you personally believe that you have been treated unfairly, then there is recourse through Human Resource (HR) policies. Check with the HR representative to see what the grievance process entails. If you are basing this opinion on the experience of others, then it is their responsibility to complain to Administration or HR. Often though, no one really knows the whole story, as personnel issues are kept confidential. Rumors can ignite and lead people astray.

If you have a concern, address it with the manager. If you are uncomfortable discussing your concerns alone, use an HR representative as a third-party facilitator. If actual inequities do occur, it is your responsibility to document these accurately and get the help you need to resolve issues.

13. *Case:* **I have high blood pressure and I am being asked to report to the employee health nurse on a weekly basis to get my blood pressure taken. Last week my blood pressure was high and I was sent home. Is this an acceptable practice?**

The Employee Health Department must work from protocols. If the organization has supported a protocol that identifies and treats hypertension in this way, then you must follow this practice. It would seem that they have your best interest at heart. It would be preferable for you to think that the employer is being preventive and wellness oriented. If the employer knew you were hypertensive and did not send you home and you have a stroke at work, then it is possible that your family could make a claim that you were placed in a harmful work condition.

Your nursing license does depend on your physical and mental ability to do the job. If your health impairs your ability to do your job functions, then to protect both patients and yourself, you should be removed from that aspect of your job until your health problems are resolved. If you still question this action, contact the state board of nursing or a nurse attorney who specializes in employment issues.

14. *Case:* **We have several fire hazards in our area but the occupational health nurse will do nothing about the problem because it would be so costly to the employer to fix. What recourse do I have?**

While the occupational health nurse has the responsibility to report these concerns, the organization's safety officer has responsibility to address them with administration. Violations of the Occupational Safety and Health Administration (OSHA) guidelines can cause hefty fines and shut down the organization, but this depends on the nature and severity of the hazard. Some may think that OSHA regulations are punitive; they are intended to save lives. This is an area where the risk of fines can outweigh the burden of costly repairs.

You also have other options. If the safety officer is not responsive or administration does not address the issue, you as an employee may contact OSHA directly about unresolved concerns. An OSHA representative is happy to talk with anyone and will send out an investigator if the situation warrants further attention. The state department that regulates healthcare facilities will also send out a safety inspector if notified. The local fire department has a prevention bureau that answers complaints as well. Once you have documented the problem with the safety officer or administration, the employee can refuse to work in the area.

15. *Case:* We have hired a considerable number of nurses for whom English is their second language. Patients/families have been complaining that they do not understand the nurses' requests and fear they do not provide good nursing care. What is the appropriate response?

This problem could be seen with increasing frequency in the coming years. The nurses should be provided with assistance with their English skills and patients/families should be assured that asking a nurse to repeat information is acceptable. Assuming you see these nurses as competent, take their concerns as opportunities to reassure them of the nurses' competence. Bring in a representative from Patient/ Visitor Relations to help both parties understand their responsibilities to keep nurse/patient communication open and clear. Document your concerns and share them with management so that they can have a perspective on the degree of the problem.

Explore options at a staff meeting to address the patient/family concerns. Bedside report is one strategy to help patients have a comfort level with the next shift's nurse and fosters a mutual understanding of the plan of care.

Partnering nurses of different cultures to work as a team, rather than isolating nurses to a group of patients, can help improve communication quickly.

16. *Case:* The hospital is paying a wage to nurse aides that does not bring them above poverty level for our area. What can I do to rectify this problem?

This is a common occurrence not isolated to nurse aides. Many people in this country are working, yet earning below the poverty level. While you may not be able to influence what wages are paid in the organization, you can advocate for a mobility program that encourages interested candidates to pursue more education, providing eligibility for higher paying positions. Health care is a supportive environment for mobility programs because skill sets tend to build on those previously acquired. Especially during this nursing shortage, employers are funding educational mobility in order to secure the licensed staff needed, but also to retain loyal and experienced employees. You can begin by talking to some of the nurse aide staff to see what their interest is in continued education and possible promotions. If there is an existing program, then encourage your colleagues to participate. If there isn't, then make the suggestion to management. You may have just created a new position for yourself.

17. *Case:* **One of the nurses on the unit is a lesbian. She has been receiving more than the average number of requests for overtime and is looking exhausted. I fear that our manager, who is suspected of disapproving of that lifestyle, is targeting her. What can I do?**

Discrimination is the practice of favoritism based on a person's race, color, religion, sex, or national origin. While sexual practices are not specifically addressed, it is considered unreasonable to base expectations on sexual orientation. Staffing guidelines in many states prohibit working unwanted overtime. No one can make someone work until they are exhausted. Even mandatory overtime cannot exceed the allowable by insurance regulations (i.e., minimum number of hours between shifts, maximum number of consecutive days/hours). The best thing you can do is share the observation with your co-worker that you notice she is tired. Ask if everything is all right or if there is anything you can do. If the co-worker denies needing assistance, then unless there is a problem with patient care, you may have no interest in this situation. If there is a problem, encourage your colleague to seek assistance through Human Resources. A case will have to be presented that the fact she is a lesbian has caused this unfair treatment. Creating a hostile work environment, one in which one worker is made to feel uncomfortable, is not condoned by any labor rules.

18. *Case:* **One of the nurses hired has six children and she cannot accept the committee work and overtime hours many of us do. She is a good clinician. What can I do to help others understand that her presence is good for our culture?**

In this nursing shortage, a good clinician is far better than no one at all. Perhaps it is time for the organization to look at its practices regarding overtime and committee work if it wants to attract more good clinicians. The coworkers questioning this nurse's contributions should be directed to the manager, as you do not have any control of this situation.

However, you could help this nurse fit in by identifying her special contributions to the unit—stability, good solid care, and a calming influence. Other nurses could be encouraged to share some of their contributions with her and get her ideas. Perhaps she might then volunteer to do literature searches at home on the computer or the typing of drafts of new policies. While she may not do the overtime, she may contribute to the overall well-being of the unit by bringing in an occasional healthy snack.

19. *Case:* **Our organization has developed core values upon which we are all evaluated. I believe in them, but many managers do not exemplify the virtues described. As a staff nurse what can I do to change our culture to manifest these values?**

Culture is determined at the top of the organization hierarchy. If you give core value awards, then nominate a manager who exemplifies the values. If your manager exemplifies the values, then discuss your concern with her/him.

As a staff nurse, your best action is to role model the values. Live and breathe the core values. People are great imitators. If you behave badly you'll be copied. If you are seen exemplifying the core values, then others will follow. If the managers are functioning against the core values, ask for a values clarification discussion so that you can be sure that everyone is operating from the same viewpoint. Propose a shared governance model for nursing practice where dialogue is openly supported.

20. *Case:* **In watching contract negotiations or even watching some of the nurses on the floor negotiate for time off, I see them use bluffing. Is not bluffing lying and therefore unethical?**

Bluffing is intentional deceit in order to show strength. Bluffing is intentionally misleading a person with a false, bold front. Since the behavior is not genuine or truthful, you could call it a form of lying. It is unfortunate that any workplace negotiations would lend themselves to bluffing. This means that there is not an environment where open and honest communication is acknowledged. Those using that degree of power over another to get what they want are not practicing good ethical behavior.

Bluffing leads management and staff to antagonistic relationships. When you are aware of this practice, it would be best to avoid participating in these situations. If you are able to point out to either or both parties how harmful this is, then you are advocating for a healthy workplace.

RESOURCES

American Academy of Pediatrics Ethics Committee. http://aapolicy.aappublic ations.org/cgi/content/full/pediatrics%3b107/1/205

American Medical Association Ethics Resource Center. http://www.ama-assn.org/ ama/pub/category/2732.html

American Nurses Association Center for Ethics and Human Rights. http://nursing world.org/ethics/

American Society for Bioethics and Humanities Core Competencies for Health Care Ethics Consultation. http://www.asbh.org/resources/publications/index.htm

Center for American Nurses. http://nursingworld.org/can/

Equal Employment Opportunity Commission. http://www.eeoc.gov/

Family and Medical Leave Act. http://www.opm.gov/oca/leave/html/fmlafact.htm

French, M., Dunlap, L., Roman, P., & Steele, P. (1996). Factors that influence the use and perceptions of employee assistance programs at six worksites. *Journal of Occupational Health Psychology, 2*(4), 313–324.

Jones, S. (2002). Employee rights, employee responsibilities, and knowledge-sharing in intelligent organizations. *Employee Responsibilities and Rights Journal, 14*(2/3), 69–78.

Keenan, J. (2002). Whistle-Blowing: A study of managerial differences. *Employee Responsibilities and Rights Journal, 14*(1), 17–32.

King, N. (2003). Electronic monitoring to promote national security impacts in workplace privacy. *Employee Responsibilities and Rights Journal, 15*(3), 127–147.

Milne, S., Blum, T., & Roman, P. (1994). Factors influencing employees' propensity to use an employee assistance program. *Personnel Psychology, 47*(1), 123–146

Occupational Safety and Health Administration. www.osha.gov

Oexman, R., Knotts, T., & Koch, J. (2002). Working while the world sleeps: A consideration of sleep and shift work design. *Employee Responsibilities and Rights Journal, 14*(4), 145–157.

Quinones, R., & Schaefer, A. (1997). The legal, ethical, and managerial implications of the neutral employment reference policy. *Employee Responsibilities and Rights Journal, 10*(2), 173–189.

Safe Staffing Guidelines—American Nurses Association. http://nursingworld.org/staffing/

United American Nurses. http://nursingworld.org/uan/

Zickers, M. (2001). *Work and unseen chronic illness: Silent voices.* London: Routledge.

Chapter 21

Ethics Committees

Barbara B. Ott

1. What is the role of the ethics committee?

The role of the ethics committee is to support education in bioethics and to improve bioethical decision making throughout the institution. This is accomplished by educating the healthcare staff, participating in policy development related to bioethical issues, developing community education programs, and supporting patients and their families as they encounter complex ethical issues related to patient care. Case consultation is an important role of the ethics committee. Cases that are troublesome to patients, families, or staff are analyzed by the committee.

2. Why does a healthcare organization need an ethics committee?

The Joint Commission on Accreditation of Healthcare Organizations (JCAHO) has established Standards on Patient Rights and Organization Ethics. All organizations that seek accreditation from JCAHO must meet the standard of addressing ethical issues. The standards were formed to ensure that patients' rights were respected and that the institution conducted its business practices in an ethical manner. The ethics committee assists in ensuring that these standards are met or exceeded. Nurses can bring cases or issues that were unable to be resolved at the unit level to the committee. Cases in which there are differences of opinion between patients or family members and the healthcare staff can be addressed by the ethics committee.

3.   Who should be on an ethics committee?

The ethics committee should be multidisciplinary because many disciplines are involved in direct patient care or institutional decisions regarding patient care. Each committee should have representatives from physicians, nurses, social workers, community members, and chaplains. It is helpful if members are selected from different religious backgrounds, ages, and races. Community members are important because they can relay the concerns of the community to the hospital and represent specific ethnic or cultural groups served by the hospital. Chaplains or clergy are especially helpful in educating staff when a patient's religious beliefs are an important factor in healthcare decision making. There is sometimes an attorney on the committee to advise the committee of Federal, state, or local laws that could influence decision making. Sometimes there is a university in the community and a faculty member who teaches healthcare ethics is a good addition to the committee.

4.   How are the members of the ethics committee selected?

Usually members are selected for the committee because they have an interest in ethical decision making. The education of the committee members is quite extensive, so the prospective member must agree to study and read materials selected by the committee. The committee chairperson usually looks for advice from the rest of the committee before selecting new members. Some committees suggest that clinicians applying for membership be mid-career level practitioners and not novice practitioners.

5.   What are the responsibilities of a member of the ethics committee?

Members of the ethics committee would be required to attend regularly scheduled meetings and occasionally attend "STAT" meetings called to address a specific case consultation or other time-sensitive issue. Members are responsible for self-education with the guidance of the committee and others. The education of the members of the ethics committee is a continuing process. It takes many months of study for a new committee member to begin to understand the ethical theory necessary to be a contributing member of the committee. Members could also be an informal representative of the committee in a liaison fashion with other departments and staff members.

6. How can I get on the ethics committee?

Most members are on the committee because they have an interest in ethical decision making. You could ask the chairperson of the committee if you could be a member. Since the education of the members takes a long time, expressing your desire to read and study ethical issues would enhance your chances of getting on the committee. Sometimes the committee will allow guests to attend a meeting or two and that may help you decide if membership on the committee is for you. The ANA (2001) *Code of Ethics for Nurses* encourages nurses to participate on ethics committees.

7. What is the difference between an institutional ethics committee, an organizational ethics committee, and an institutional review board?

An institutional ethics committee is concerned with ethical aspects of the institution. If the institution is a hospital, the committee is concerned with the ethical aspects of patient care and educating the staff of the hospital to such issues as DNR orders, privacy issues, or the informed consent process. An organizational ethics committee is concerned about the ethical aspects of organizational decision making. For instance, if there are several hospitals in an organization, each hospital could have an institutional ethics committee and then there would be one committee with representatives from each institutional committee serving on an organizational ethics committee. The issues of importance to the organizational ethics committee could be things such as: Who are we buying our supplies from, and why? Are the prices charged for services appropriate? Is the community well served by the institution? Are there any conflicts of interests that should be examined? Are the institution's resources allocated in an appropriate manner? An institutional review board is a committee required by the Federal Department of Health and Human Services that is designed to protect human subjects who participate in research. The committee reviews research proposals and monitors ongoing research to safeguard the rights of human subjects.

8. When is an ethics consultation indicated?

An ethics consultation is indicated when there are differences among family members, between the nurse and the physician, between physician and physician, or between physician and patient/family. A consultation is also indicated when an individual believes that there is an ethical dilemma that is not being addressed, such as a case where advance directives are not being followed. Nurses can bring a case before the ethics committee and most hospital policies say that anyone can bring a case before the committee. A consultation is also indicated when a nurse or nurses are having difficulty following a hospital policy as currently written.

9. What types of cases are brought to the ethics committee?

Cases brought to the ethics committee may involve treatment decisions in individual cases such as withholding or withdrawing therapy, refusal or discontinuation of life-sustaining therapy, or evaluating decision-making capacity. Many policy issues are brought to the committee such as the following issues: confidentiality or privacy policies, informed consent, DNR policies, pain management, who is admitted to the ICU, or HIV testing.

10. What happens when a particular case is brought to the ethics committee for consultation?

The case is discussed including the following:

1. the identification of the medical problems

2. diagnoses, prognoses, goals of treatment, recommendations for further treatment or care

3. reasonable alternatives available

4. the patient's ability to make decisions

5. the presence of a surrogate decision maker

6. the preferences of the decision makers

7. complicating interests (e.g., is the patient pregnant, does the case involve unusually scarce resources, is there family disagreement, or is there disagreement between the healthcare team and the patient or surrogate)

8. the moral problems

9. policies and ethical standards or guidelines from professional specialty groups

10. similar cases from the literature

11. alternative solutions

All committee members and guests are asked to participate in the discussion; the ethically acceptable alternatives for resolving the case are identified; and these alternatives are made known to those involved in the case.

11. How are decisions made on the ethics committee? Do committee members vote?

The committee discusses issues in depth. During that discussion different options are discussed and analyzed. The goal is to reach a consensus opinion of the committee. However, occasionally there could be one or two dissenting opinions. If there is no consensus, the issue probably needs more attention from the committee and future meetings on the topic would be scheduled.

12. What should the ethics committee write on the chart after a consultation?

The committee should write several things on the patient's chart after an ethics consultation including: date and time of consultation, individual requesting the consultation, summary of the reason for the consultation, sources of information used in the consultation, identification of ethical issues, brief discussion of ethical analysis of the case, and recommendations of the ethically acceptable alternatives.

13. Do physicians treating patients have to do what the ethics committee says?

No, physicians are not required to do what the ethics committee recommends. The committee makes recommendations to physicians usually in the form of a list of ethically acceptable alternatives from which to choose. Usually, physicians take the recommendations of the ethics committee seriously and choose one of the recommendations.

14. What are the rules or standards for ethics committees?

The American Society for Bioethics and Humanities has established Core Competencies for Health Care Ethics Consultation (www.asbh.org). These competencies describe skills and standards necessary for an ethics committee to do healthcare ethics consultation. These skills include: the ability to identify and analyze the values in conflict, to identify the agents involved, to ensure concerned parties have their voices heard, to access relevant knowledge in the law, policy, and professional codes, and to identify and justify morally acceptable options. The standards require some members of the committee to have advanced skills and others to have basic skills in several areas of ethical analysis.

15. Should the nurse caring for the patient attend an ethics consultation meeting about a patient in his/her care?

Yes, the nurse caring for the patient should attend the ethics consultation meeting. The nurse can add valuable knowledge about the patient's response to care and treatments. Many patients and families communicate well with the nurse and that information can be valuable for decision making.

16. Can the patient and/or family attend the ethics consultation meeting?

The patient and/or the family or other surrogate decision makers should be invited to attend the consultation meeting. They have a stake in the deliberations and can best articulate their goals and values. Those arranging the ethics consultation meeting should accommodate the availability of the patient and/or family. There should also be a person assigned to the family to act as an advocate, to make certain that the family understands what is being said, and has ample opportunities to speak and have all of their questions and concerns addressed.

17. Can the ethics committee be sued?

Yes, the ethics committee can be sued for negligence or for violating the rights of patients during case consultations; however, this is exceedingly rare. Members of the ethics committee should be concerned about the legal consequences of consultation services, but this concern should not direct case consultations.

18. How is an ethics consultation service different from an ethics committee?

An institutional ethics committee is usually an internal committee, comprised of members employed by the institution with a few from outside the institution. An ethics consultation service is usually an external or "free standing" consultation service (not connected to a hospital or university) that offers its services for a fee. Sometimes this service is offered by a single, independent ethics consultant.

19. Is a single, independent ethics consultant better than an ethics committee?

No. In fact, in my opinion, it is worse. It is better to have several different voices on an ethics committee, all analyzing a case or policy rather than a single and independent ethics consultant. We all value things differently and a single consultant can more easily place his/her values on others.

20. Does the ethics committee change hospital policies?

Ethics committees influence changes in hospital policies after careful review of the existing policies. The committee makes recommendations to different departments, committees, or to the board of directors. These recommendations can eventually result in changes in hospital policies.

21. What do I do if I have an ethics problem in the middle of the night?

Each ethics committee should have a policy or procedure that directs staff to someone to call in the middle of the night if there is an ethical concern. Many committees generate an "on call" list that is available to nursing supervisors, telephone operators, or administrators on call. An ethics consultation can be generated in the middle of the night if a particular case cannot wait until the morning. It is important that all physicians and nurses on duty at night are aware of how to "get the ball rolling" on an ethics consultation in the middle of the night.

RESOURCES

American Nurses Association. (2001). *Code of ethics for nurses with interpretive statements.* Washington, DC: American Nurses Publishing.

Fletcher, J., & Spencer, E. (1997). Ethics services in health care organizations. In J. Fletcher, P. Lombardo, M. Marshall, & F. Miller (Eds.), *Introduction to clinical ethics* (2nd ed., pp. 257–286). Hagerstown, MD: University Publishing Group, Inc.

Joint Commission on Accreditation of Healthcare Organizations (JCAHO). (2003). *2003 Hospital accreditation standards.* Oakbrook Terrace, IL: Author.

Monagle, J. F., & Thomasma, D. C. (1998). *Health care ethics.* Gaithersburg, MD: Aspen Publishers, Inc.

Part 6

The Mix of Culture and Religion With Ethics

Though no book can describe the tapestry of human experience, these two chapters address the religious and cultural differences that could create misunderstanding leading to inferior nursing care. The answers point out the different views of the same event, whether it is caretaking, informed consent, or dying. The purpose is not to stereotype, but to help nurses examine the issues by generalizing. Generalizing begins with an assumption about a group, but leads to seeking further information about whether this assumption fits the individual patient. The hope is that you will find these chapters a step in your journey in learning what mysteries the different realities of religions and cultures unfamiliar to us hold.

Chapter 22

Religion and Ethics

Syvil S. Burke

1. What are some of the ethical issues a clinician will have to confront because of a patient's religious preference?

Religious beliefs form a part of one's identity as a person. It is important for a clinician to understand that respecting the exercise of these beliefs is a part of respecting the individual as a person. The greatest dilemma for the clinician is when respecting the importance of a patient's religious beliefs has a bearing on decisions about care. When a patient's views are grounded in religious teachings and convictions, attempts to dissuade could be interpreted as attempts to impose the healthcare professional's beliefs on the patient. Religious restrictions and convictions can affect treatment options, provision of life-sustaining therapies, timing of therapies, and end-of-life care. All of these raise ethical issues for the clinician. The clinician has an obligation to ensure that communication occurs with the patient and family to ensure that an informed choice is made in the context of religious justification for refusal of care or determination of type of care to be provided. A patient or family's right to practice the mandates of their religion does not translate into an automatic obligation on the part of the clinician to oblige, especially if the restrictions are morally unacceptable to the clinician. The clinician, however, does have a responsibility to respect the right of the patient to his/her religious preference and to develop a plan of care plan that incorporates this respect or to arrange for the transition of the patient's care to another healthcare provider.

2. What do you do when a patient asks you to pray with him and you are not religious?

As a member of the healthcare team your focus is to promote the patient's well-being by assisting in the development of a plan of care to include treatment options and goals. Prayer may be important to the patient and a desired intervention. A healthcare provider can limit involvement in this type of activity, if he does not believe in prayer or has no desire to pray. However, all attempts should be made to assist patients with their requests for prayer. Hospital chaplains and those involved in clinical pastoral education programs are spiritual resources for patients. In addition, the assistance of other members of the healthcare team who feel comfortable in praying with patients is also welcomed.

3. Is it ethical to discuss topics of a spiritual nature with a patient?

Patients are emotionally, physically, and spiritually vulnerable. Life events such as physical illness, suffering, death, and birth can have significant spiritual meaning for them. Patients desire to establish trust with the members of the healthcare team. As a result there may be a significant need or desire to discuss topics of a spiritual nature with members of the team. It is ethical to discuss topics of a spiritual nature with a patient as long as such discussions do not attempt to lead the patient in a different spiritual direction from where the patient desires. Therefore, it is unethical for a clinician to create a situation where the clinician's own interests, beliefs, or values are inflicted on the patients.

4. What do you do when a physician communicates that he cannot withdraw support/treatment from a patient because he views that as murder?

If a patient's physician objects to the direction of care, because of a religious or moral perspective, it can be viewed as conscientious objection. This objection can be accommodated but patient rights must also be respected. The physician is not obligated to proceed with the withdrawal of support/ treatment, but is obligated to arrange for a transfer of care to a physician who would be able to do so. The only interests of the provider that should ever enter and influence the decision process would be those that affect the medical interest of the patient.

5. What do you do if a family is unwilling to consent to withdrawal of support for their loved one because they are waiting for a miracle?

If a patient's prognosis is poor or if further treatment is futile, it is imperative that open and frank discussions occur to include the patient's clinical status and prognosis in language understandable to the family. This discussion needs to include the reasoning that underlies any recommendations that treatment be withheld or withdrawn. Even with such discussions, clinicians and families often find themselves at an impasse when there is nothing else that can be done medically. Families often desire to wait for spiritual intervention to manifest itself in answers to prayers and miracles. It is important for the team to clarify the religious perspective or personal beliefs that have led to their refusal.

It is also important to determine whether the family's refusal represents their knowledge of the patient's wishes or rather their own interpretation of what the interests of the patient would have been. Resources such as ethics committee representatives, social workers, and chaplains all are beneficial in assisting the family and the medical team in such discussions. With continued family refusal, physicians are under no obligation to accede to family demands for continued treatment if it is not in accord with the accepted standard of care under the circumstances. No one has a legally supportable right other than to receive whatever care is given according to accepted medical standards.

6. *Case:* A patient is very depressed and is suicidal as evidenced by all my assessments. She is also a very religious person. What are the various religious views on suicide that I can use to support her in not killing herself?

A major area of agreement for all religions is the sanctity of life. Since most religions view a human as not the creator of his/her self, the life of the individual is not his/hers to extinguish. Suicide is viewed as self-murder and there is a spiritual consequence to suicide. Suicide is viewed as a crime against the soul and considered an unforgivable sin. All major religions raise questions about the outcome of the soul of a person who commits this act. Therefore, it is important to help the patient understand that suicide will not help her to escape life but may get her in a far worse situation when she thinks of what may happen to her after death.

7. Are the wishes of Jehovah's Witnesses to not have blood transfusions to be honored at all times?

For Jehovah's Witnesses, biblical teachings prohibiting the eating and drinking of blood support their refusal to accept blood transfusions. A transfusion symbolizes drinking another person's blood and represents a flagrant sin. It is believed that blood once removed from the body should be disposed of and not transfused into another person's body.

Decision-making capacity is the patient's ability to consider the factors relevant to a specific decision and his/her personal values and to engage in autonomous decision making. A Jehovah's Witness has the moral and legal right to consent to, or to refuse any treatment intervention, including blood transfusions. Even if the decision is to risk death rather than receive a transfusion, it is the patient's right if it is made in an informed and voluntary manner. It is unethical to give Jehovah's Witnesses blood products against their wishes.

When there is no advance knowledge of whether a patient is a Jehovah's Witness, and there is an emergent need for a blood transfusion, it is appropriate to presume that the patient would want the blood transfusion. However, once it is clear that the patient has decision-making capacity and understands options and their consequences, then the patient's choice should be respected.

If healthcare team members find it morally unacceptable to comply with the patient's wishes, or if it is believed that the medical or surgical treatments could not be provided without the possibility of the need for blood products, then there is an obligation to transfer the patient to another healthcare team or to another healthcare facility to provide the care and respect the patient's wishes for bloodless surgery.

8. In caring for Jehovah's Witnesses, am I to assume that they will refuse all blood products?

Jehovah's Witnesses believe that it is a violation of God's law to accept whole blood, plasma, platelets, red cells, and white cells. However, the trend in recent years has been to allow more blood products. The use of fractions of the primary blood components is acceptable. The separate components of plasma such as globulin, fibrinogens, and albumin are permitted. In addition, the use of hemoglobin is accepted since it is fractionated from red blood cells.

The Associated Jehovah's Witnesses for Reform on Blood has recently been formed and is composed of a diverse group of Witnesses from many countries, professions, and advocacy groups. Over time we may continue to see additional steps toward the acceptance of a greater number of blood products.

9. **Case: A Roman Catholic patient wants to have a child very badly and is considering in vitro insemination. She thinks that it is prohibited by the Church. Is that true?**

The Roman Catholic Church condemns any form of artificial method used for conception. The use of another person, as signified by the use of donated sperm or ovum or a surrogate, is considered immoral. This represents betrayal of the spouses' rights to become parents only through each other. In addition, the child's right to be born of a father and mother known to it and bound by marriage is affected. Even if the artificial technique involves only the married couple, the Church views the procreative act as dissociated from the expected sexual act and, therefore, immoral. Procreation in this sense would have been influenced by technology. For the Church, the two principles undergirding the reproduction process are: (1) the possibility of procreation and (2) the love union. The church only respects the link between the conjugal love of parents and the right of a child to be the fruit of the specific act of this conjugal love.

10. **Can a hospital chaplain perform last rites on a Catholic patient if there is no priest available?**

The performance of last rites has changed over the years. In the past last rites were associated with death and performed the last day of life only by a priest. Changes in health care have ushered in the need for different approaches to the pastoral care needs of the sick and dying. The Catholic Church now offers several rites or sacraments that are appropriate for the sick, the dying, and the dead. These sacraments are: reconciliation, anointing, communion, and confirmation. The sacraments of reconciliation and anointing require the presence of a priest. They are for the living and meant to bring healing. If someone has died, there will be no anointing. Prayers are offered for the dead. Anyone can offer prayers and the presence of a priest is not required. Since the focus at the time of death is on praying for patients, a hospital chaplain can perform this rite. A priest or a lay minister may administer communion. There is a special form of communion for the dying called Viaticum, which can be delivered by a chaplain. Last, for those who have never been confirmed and find themselves near death, a priest is needed for this sacrament.

11. A Jewish patient's son has just committed suicide. Though I understand she is upset, she is refusing to make funeral arrangements. Is this a typical response to suicide in the Jewish religion?

For Judaism, God owns everything, including our bodies. God lends our bodies to us for the duration of our lives and we return them to God when we die. Consequently, neither men nor women have the right to govern their own bodies as they will. Jews have a duty to preserve their own lives. They are commanded not only to do virtually anything necessary to save their own lives; they are also bound by positive obligation to take steps to save the lives of others.

Therefore, Jews do not make funeral arrangements for anyone who has committed suicide, nor do they mourn for him or eulogize. However, they do stand in line to greet others who would normally mourn him/her, recite the mourner's blessing, and participate in other activities, which honor the living.

12. I know that in the Jewish religion there is no prohibition against organ transplants. Are they allowed to accept transplantation of genes?

The use of genetic testing and engineering as a tool for combating genetically based diseases is strongly endorsed by a broad spectrum of Jewish opinion, including opinions by the Orthodox quarter. Orthodoxy accepts gene transplants as an analog of organ transplants. The Jewish tradition affirms that humankind was created in the image of God and while there is no law that precludes tampering with the human being's DNA, it truly does preclude tampering with a human being's basic humanity.

Humans are composed of genes, energy, and the spirit of God. All govern and play a role in our circumstances, or choices, and our actions. Behavior may be genetically regulated, hormonally expressed, and environmentally mediated and modified, but the overriding mechanism of will, the veto power of autonomous free choice coupled with the power of divine, is always with us. There is general agreement among rabbis that the legitimacy of human intervention to affect cure extends to procedures within the womb as well. When used in this therapeutic way, genetic engineering is seen as a blessing.

13. How do I accommodate a hospitalized Muslim who desires to fast during Ramadan?

Ramadan is the Muslim holy month in which Muslims fast from just before sunrise to sunset each day. Ramadan fasting is obligatory for the healthy adult, but when fasting might affect the health of the individual or when one is sick, Islam exempts him/her from fasting. However, a significant number of patients, for their own reasons, decide to observe the fast. It is imperative in cases of illness that Muslim patients who desire to fast do so under medical supervision. Adjustments in the medication regimen and treatment plan would assist the patient in meeting his/her religious need. However, patient safety is the priority. If the patient develops symptoms or if his/her health is adversely affected, the fast must be discontinued immediately.

14. A Muslim patient requests that his bed be repositioned so that he can pray. How should I respond?

It is a requirement for every Muslim to perform five obligatory prayers per day. All prayers must be said while facing in the direction of Mecca, the location of the first house ever built for the worship of one God. By facing Mecca there is unity and order in prayer. The patient's right to practice the mandates of his religion is not unlimited. If the repositioning of the bed will bring harm to the patient or interfere with the ability of the healthcare team to provide care, the first priority must be patient care. If, on the other hand, it is possible to accommodate the patient's request, the bed should be repositioned to acknowledge respect for the patient's right to his religious beliefs.

15. Does the Muslim ban on the consumption of pork refer to medications also?

Muslims are told in the Qur'an not to eat pork or pork by-products. In addition, any medication that contains any derivative of pork is strictly forbidden. A medication containing pork by-products can only be administered if it is a lifesaving necessity or when a non-pork alternative is not available.

16. How do you respond to a Christian Scientist patient who wants to be discharged from the hospital because God has revealed to her that she is healed?

Christian Scientists believe that God has the power to heal illness and all forms of evil. Christian Scientists normally choose prayer alone for healing for themselves. However, an individual is always free to choose whatever form of treatment or care he/she believes will best answer his/her need.

Every hospitalized patient with decision-making capacity, or the ability to consider the factors relevant to a specific decision and his/her personal values and to engage in autonomous decision making, has the right to self-determination. Therefore, if a Christian Scientist has chosen to come to the hospital for care but then wants to be discharged because she believes she has been healed, she has that right. The healthcare provider is only obligated to disclose to the patient all reasonable information regarding his/her condition and needed care. It would be unethical to not respond to the patient's request for discharge. One cannot impose treatment on a competent person who does not desire to be treated.

17. *Case:* The mother of a Buddhist patient states that it would be considered murder to not insert a PEG tube for feeding. Is this true?

In the case of a patient in a persistent vegetative state who has not been declared dead on the criteria of brainstem death, the provision of food and hydration should be continued. There would, however, be no requirement to treat subsequent complications, for example pneumonia or other infections, by administering antibiotics.

In Buddhist jurisprudence, the key ingredient in murder is the intention to cause death; whether the death results from an act of omission is of little importance.

If a person sought the death of another and brought it about by depriving the person of food, he would be just as guilty as if he had used a knife.

On these grounds, Buddhism would hold that a physician has a duty to act for the well-being of his/her patients, and that to bring about a patient's death by deliberate omission would be morally as grave as causing the death by a deliberate act. For Buddhism all persons, regardless of their physical condition, are worthy of compassion. Buddhism stresses the need for universal, as opposed to selected, benevolence and to exclude patients in a persistent vegetative state from this care would be arbitrary and unjust.

18. I understand that Buddhism does not support abortion, yet I read that the abortion rate in Japan is higher than in the United States. Please help me understand this.

Buddhism takes the stand that the right to life for all beings must be respected. The formation of a child's mind and body is said to begin in the womb. In fact, in Buddhist scriptures, 5 of the 10 stages between life and death occur inside the womb. Buddhists believe that life is produced in the womb at conception. They also do not believe in embryo research because it involves the destruction of human embryos.

One of the factors that seem to have played an important role in shaping Japanese attitudes toward abortion is the traditional view of the fetus. Central to Japanese perspectives on abortion is the concept of *mizuko* or culture "waterchild." This is the name given to the fetus. Traditional Japanese culture conceptualizes the fetus as a being whose existence is fluid and indeterminate. A fetus is thought to exist partly in a human world and partly in the spirit. It can be argued that abortion does not involve the killing of a "full" human being since the spirit is not yet completely committed to human existence. In terms of this belief, abortion can be seen not so much as the destruction of life as its postponement, a nudging of the fetus back into the world of the gods from where it came. However, many Japanese Buddhists remain ambivalent about abortion.

19. If a patient is a member of the Adventist church what should I be aware of in his/her care?

Adventists accept the Bible literally and believe that evidence of salvation is keeping of the Commandments. The body is considered the temple of

God and must be kept healthy. Therefore, most Adventists adhere to a vegetarian diet and avoid alcohol, coffee, and tea. There are no restrictions on medications, blood, or blood products. The only restriction on surgical procedures could occur when a patient might refuse an intervention on Friday evening and Saturday (Sabbath). The pastor or elders may come to pray and anoint an ill person with oil. They believe that healing is accomplished through medical intervention, as well as divine healing.

20. **Case: A patient is Native American and I find the chanting and praying in his room very interesting. When this occurs I am not sure if I should stay, though I have not been asked to leave. What should I do?**

The patient and family members would consider it rude to ask a nurse to leave, so it is best if you give them privacy. You could also help the hospital chaplain to not pray out loud when he/she is with the patient because out of respect the chaplain would likely not be asked by the patient or family to pray in silence. The medicine man or woman is seen as very important in assisting in the healing process. This individual would probably be present and introduced as a cousin or uncle, rather than a spiritual leader. It is believed that the medicine man or woman has the capacity to heal through prayers, ceremony, and spiritual powers given by ancestors.

Native Americans also use sacred instruments such as a medicine bag, sand, and sage sticks. Since these instruments are considered sacred, you should not touch them without permission. Usually family members or friends are the individuals who will move these instruments of healing. It is also improper to ask about the contents of the medicine bag that the individual usually wears around his/her neck.

RESOURCES

Doyle, D. (2002). Blood transfusions and the Jehovah's Witness patient. *American Journal of Therapeutics, 9*(5), 417–424.

Keeft, P. (2001). *Catholic Christianity. A complete catechism of Catholic beliefs based on the catechism of the Catholic church.* Ft. Collins, CO: Ignatius Press.

Keown, D. (2001). *Buddhism and bioethics.* New York: Palgrave.

Kirkwood, N. (1999). *Hospital handbook on multiculturalism and religion: Practical guidelines for health care workers.* Harrisburg, PA: Morehouse Publishing.

Lipson, J., Dibble, S., & Minarick, P. (1996). *Culture and nursing care: A pocket guide.* San Francisco, CA: UCSF Nursing Press.

PBS Religion and Ethics News weekly. www.pbs.org/wnet/religionandethics/welcome.html

Robinson, G. (2000). *Essential Judaism: A complete guide to beliefs, customs and rituals.* New York: Simon and Schuster.

Chapter 23

Culture and Ethics

Joyce Bedoian

1. What does acculturation mean? How does this definition affect those seeking and providing health care?

According to the *Merriam-Webster Dictionary*, acculturation means

1. cultural modification of an individual, group, or people by adapting to or borrowing traits from another culture; *also* a merging of cultures as a result of prolonged contact

2. the process by which a human being acquires the culture of a particular society from infancy.

It is difficult for those of a different culture to place their trust in Western medicine. Traditional healers and lay people have been providing care in many cultures for hundreds of years. Many elders seek formalized health care as a last resort, often at the urging of younger family members or friends. For the elderly, Western customs and language are very foreign and they find it difficult to navigate the Western medical health system. As the definition suggests, individuals adapt or borrow from other cultures; they do not abandon their native culture. This makes it important for healthcare providers to be aware of the beliefs of others and be prepared to honor those beliefs.

2. African Americans have a very low enrollment in organ donation and hospice care. Why is that?

A few reasons are mistrust of the medical community, fear of premature death, and fear that their organs would only be given to white recipients. Many issues of mistrust also surround the use of hospice services. People from many ethnic groups believe it is the family's responsibility to care for dying. Through organizations like Minority Organ Tissue Transplant Education Program (MOTTEP), minorities are becoming aware of the need for donation and the number of donors is increasing. Education about hospice services is being organized in churches and community centers in many ethnic communities.

3. How do Chinese and Western cultures differ in beliefs related to disease, treatment, and death?

Chinese medicine views health as a balance with nature and the cosmos. When someone is ill there is an interruption or blockage in their "Qi" (pronounced chee) or energy flow. This Qi is similar to the Western concept of electric energy. Qi flows through channels throughout the body. A Chinese practitioner might use acupuncture to open up or redirect the Qi. Treatment is based on a holistic approach with special emphasis on mind and spirit. Death occurs when Qi dissipates. Western medicine considers the body a combination of parts and systems that need to be repaired. Organisms cause illness and can be destroyed with medications, surgery, or radiation. Death is considered a failure of treatment.

Traditional Chinese healers give credit to Western medicine for advances in trauma and acute care. Traditional Chinese medicine may be better suited for chronic illness and preventive care.

4. Our society values autonomy. Who is the decision maker in other cultures?

People from other cultures tend to rely on the elders or the eldest male in the family to guide decision making. If a patient is reluctant to give consent for a treatment or wants to wait for explanations about disease and treatment until family members are present, he/she is exercising autonomy.

5. Many of my foreign patients don't speak English. Is it okay to let a family member translate?

It is not appropriate to let a family member translate unless other means to find a translator have been exhausted. Aside from confidentiality issues, family members often interpret rather than translate to protect the patient from embarrassment. If a family member is used to translate, pay attention to the age and gender as this may affect what information is relayed. A younger family member may feel uncomfortable asking an elder certain questions. A woman may not feel comfortable discussing reproductive issues in front of a male family member. Before using a family member try one of the telephone translation services. It is likely that the institution subscribes to a service such as AT&T.

6. **I notice a big difference in how people from different cultures respond to pain. How is pain viewed in other cultures?**

Most people experience pain sensations in similar ways. How they respond and express their discomfort varies depending on their socialization to pain. People from some cultures are stoic and consider pain a fact of illness. They are appreciative of care and feel disrespectful asking for medications. People from other cultures are more vocal. Fear of addiction is also another reason patients may refuse pain medication. Scarcity of medication in some countries makes patients reluctant to ask for pain medication as they do not want to use more than their share of medication for fear of depriving someone in more distress of treatment. Some people view injections as being a stronger form of pain medication and may not realize that forms of oral analgesia are equally as effective.

7. **Why do women from other cultures wait until their breast cancer is very advanced to come in for treatment?**

Women with breast lesions are not the only type of patient who might present in later stages of illness. A general mistrust of the Western medical system, lack of finances to pay for care, or fear of deportation may contribute to patients' waiting to seek care. Modesty and discomfort talking about personal appearance may also be reasons. It is often family members who recognize a problem and encourage the patient to seek care. Remaining non-judgmental and supportive will put the patient at ease and facilitate entry into the healthcare system.

8. **Why did a Sikh family get so upset when we shaved their son's hair before his brain surgery?**

Unshorn hair and beard are part of a Sikh's "outer badges" that reflect the Sikh's military history. Many cultures believe that long thick hair is a sign of health—much like the biblical tale of Samson, who lost his strength when his hair was cut. Native Americans also believe that cutting a person's hair will cause him/her harm. If the hair must be shaved or cut, the family may want to bring in a "medicine pouch" and place it near the patient's body to promote healing.

9. I see a lot of bruises on Asian children when they are sick. Are they punished for being ill?

Coin rubbing is a traditional form of healing in Asian cultures. A coin or spoon is heated or dipped in oil and the affected area of the body is rubbed until a raised, red mark appears. The raised, red mark is believed to mean the illness has risen to the surface of the body and will then be able to leave the body. Another form of traditional healing that will leave marks on the body is cupping. A glass is heated and placed on the affected area of the body. A vacuum is created and the glass is removed. The treatment leaves a raised, round mark. Cupping is used in many cultures including Asia, Latin America, and many parts of Europe and is even taught in the United States in homeopathic and other alternative healing programs.

10. Sometimes it is not possible to allow a cultural healer to see a patient in the hospital. What are the possible ramifications for the patient?

Shaman and other traditional healers have been treating illness and infirmity in other cultures for hundreds of years. It is important to realize that when people from other cultures seek Western medical care, they may also continue care by their traditional healer. They are often uncomfortable with Western medical practice but are seeking care because they have been encouraged to do so by a family member or friend or because traditional treatments have failed. It is important to be aware of what treatments have been tried by the traditional healer and if that treatment is continuing in order to know whether it may interfere with Western medical treatment. Faith and spirituality are important components of health in other cultures and denying a patient access to his/her traditional healer may cause him/her not to accept Western medical care or take away his/her hope for cure.

11. I am finding managing the symptoms of a Mexican American patient very difficult. Is there a prohibition against

reporting pain, shortness of breath, diarrhea, and other symptoms?

Mexican Americans prize inner control and self-endurance. Expression of pain is socially acceptable in women; however, stoicism is common in men. They also believe that when oxygen is required, that there must be something very wrong with them, so they have a tendency not to report shortness of breath. Some believe diarrhea is beneficial purging and may not agree with the use of medications to stop it. Depression is seen as a sign of weakness and embarrassment to the family, although it is the most common response to stress in Mexican Americans. Mexican Americans may seek biomedical health care for severe symptoms while using folk healing measures to deal with chronic symptoms.

12. Does postmortem care differ in other cultures?

Yes! For example, Hmongs believe in reincarnation and believe the body must be whole for the next life so will refuse organ donation or autopsy. Orthodox Jews believe the body must be whole for resurrection and may ask that amputated limbs, organs removed during surgery, and bloody clothing be wrapped with the body for burial. Many Muslims believe the body belongs to God and potential disfigurement from autopsy or organ donation should be avoided. The body must be returned as it was created. It is important to be aware of a patient and family's beliefs after death so customs can be observed before and during postmortem care.

13. If I see a female who has been circumcised, do I need to report that as abuse?

Female circumcision is illegal in this country. It is still practiced in many African countries. If you encounter a woman who has had genital-altering surgery it is important to remain non-judgmental and supportive. It is possible that the surgery was done in another country. If the procedure was done in this country, the woman should be given the option of reporting the event.

14. Why do families ask us not to tell the patient his/her diagnosis? Aren't we obligated to tell every patient his/her diagnosis?

In the Hispanic culture, for example, a serious or terminal diagnosis is withheld from the patient because it is believed the stress of knowing the diagnosis will interfere with the person's ability to heal. The "right to know" is an American concept tied to the principle of autonomy. Remember the patient has a right *not* to know. It is important to determine the patient and family's desire for information upon admission.

15. I am getting very frustrated. I notice people from other cultures are always late for appointments. Don't they understand we have to keep a schedule and these late arrivals put us behind?

Many people from other countries operate on a "present time" orientation (time relevant to a specific situation) rather than a clock. In many languages the word for time does not exist. They feel it rude to interrupt one activity to start another one. If they come from an area where agriculture is the main economy, they use the sun and weather conditions to determine their day. If they are from a European country, lunch and dinner times vary: lunch is late afternoon and dinner can be as late as 10:00 p.m. It is important to stress the importance of time, but to realize that these habits are difficult to change.

16. I find that many people from other countries don't look me in the eye when they speak. Are they lying or trying to hide something?

In many cultures avoiding eye contact is a sign of respect. In Middle Eastern countries, eye contact between males and females is considered a sexual invitation.

17. *Case:* I was taking care of an Arab patient who had his right hand in a cast after a trauma. He wouldn't feed himself or participate in his own care despite having a perfectly useful left hand. Why wouldn't he use his good left hand to participate in his care?

In the Arab tradition, the right hand is used to eat and the left hand is used to clean after going to the bathroom. Food is eaten out of communal bowls in many Middle Eastern countries and it is important to keep the right hand clean.

18. I find Native Americans reluctant to discuss advance directives. Why is that?

Native Americans believe goodness, harmony, and a positive attitude promote good health and healing. Discussing advance directives and death goes against this philosophy. Native Americans also tend to be oriented in the present and this negative discussion of the future has no place in their culture.

19. *Case:* A Hispanic daughter is already caring for her aunt at home. Now her family wants her to care for her father, too. Don't they understand this could be too much for her?

Providing care for a family member at home is a standard in many cultures. Many cultures are paternalistic in their beliefs that women marry and raise families while men work outside the home. It is important to keep the family unit intact and that often means that the care of the ill or elderly falls on an unmarried woman. In the Hispanic culture it would be considered a daughter's duty, especially if she is unmarried, and a sign of disrespect if she refused.

20. A Filipino patient is unwilling to discuss anything about her care without a family member present. Is this typical?

Filipinos are typically shy and awkward in unfamiliar surroundings. They demonstrate respect to their elders and authority figures. It is important to include close family members because this is a very family-oriented culture.

Sometimes three family generations live in a household. The father or eldest son acts as the family spokesperson; however, decisions are usually made by the entire family. Men are expected to make decisions or arrangements while women act as the primary bedside care providers, regardless of whether the patient is male or female.

RESOURCES

Crow, K., Matheson, L., & Steed, A. (2000). Informed consent and truth telling: Cultural directions for healthcare providers. *Journal of Nursing Administration,* 3(30), 148–152.

Galanti, G. A. (1997). *Caring for patients from different cultures.* Philadelphia: University of Pennsylvania Press.

Lawrence, P., & Rozmus, C. (2002). Culturally sensitive care of the Muslim patient. *Journal of Transcultural Nursing,* 3(12), 228–233.

Minority Organ Tissue Transplant Education Program (National MOTTEP). http://www.nationalmottep.org

Transcultural Nursing Society. http://www.tcns.org

United Network for Organ Sharing. http://www.unos.org

Appendix

ANA Code of Ethics for Nurses

1. The nurse, in all professional relationships, practices with compassion and respect for the inherent dignity, worth, and uniqueness of every individual, unrestricted by considerations of social or economic status, personal attributes, or the nature of health problems.

2. The nurse's primary commitment is to the patient, whether an individual, family group, or community.

3. The nurse promotes, advocates for, and strives to protect the health, safety, and rights of the patient.

4. The nurse is responsible and accountable for individual nursing practice and determines the appropriate delegation of tasks consistent with the nurse's obligation to provide optimum patient care.

5. The nurse owes the same duties to self as to others, including the responsibility to preserve integrity and safety, to maintain competence, and to continue personal and professional growth.

6. The nurse participates in establishing, maintaining, and improving health care environments and conditions of employment conducive to the provision of quality health care and consistent with the values of the profession through individual and collective action.

7. The nurse participates in the advancement of the profession through contributions to practice, education, administration, and knowledge development.

8. The nurse collaborates with other health professionals and the public in promoting community, national, and international efforts to meet health needs.

9. The profession of nursing, as represented by associations and their members, is responsible for articulating nursing values, for maintaining the integrity of the profession and its practice, and for shaping social policy.

Source: American Nurses Association. (2001). *Code of Ethics for Nurses With Interpretive Statements.* Washington, DC: American Nurses Publishing. Available with interpretive statements at www.ana.org. Reprinted with permission.

Index

Nursing Home Ethics
Everyday Issues Affecting Residents with Dementia
Bethel Ann Powers, RN, PhD

"...represents a significant new direction in consideration of the ethical issues surrounding dementia care. The case material is pertinent and compelling. This is an important contribution to the literature in the area."
—**Jaber F. Gubrium,** PhD, Professor and Chair Department of Sociology, University of Missouri

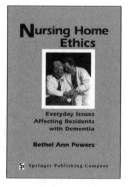

"...an important, well-organized, practical, and lucid treatment of ethical issues that arise in nursing homes. Attention to dementia makes this book an important addition to the small literature on ethics and long-term care and a must-read for members of nursing home ethics committees. The cases are vivid and plausible, and the format for discussing them particularly useful so that professionals can try to solve problems keeping in mind the needs and interests of all parties concerned, including residents with and without Alzheimer's disease, family members, and staff."
—**Rosalie A. Kane ,** DSW, School of Public Health, University of Minnesota

Powers provides a comprehensive and thoughtful examination of the ethical issues that arise in long term care. The first two chapters set the stage by exploring the pre-nursing home experiences of families living with dementia and, in contrast, how residents and family members experience life in the nursing home.

The chapters contain detailed hypothetical cases that include questions, possible actions, and insightful commentary to illustrate practical approaches to understanding ethical issues. The book also contains a useful Appendix focused on creating a Nursing Home Ethics Committee.

2003   224pp   0-8261-1964-6   softcover

11 West 42nd Street, New York, NY 10036-8002 • Fax: 212-941-7842
Order Toll-Free: 877-687-7476 • Order On-line: www.springerpub.com

Smart Nursing

How to Create a Positive Work Environment that Empowers and Retains Nurses

June Fabre, MBA, RNC

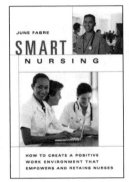

Smart Nursing describes practical techniques that every nurse, manager, and organization can use to restore patient safety, reduce nurse turnover, and stimulate realistic healthcare solutions. Solid data from business and healthcare sources are used throughout. The management practices described combine the promotion of six basic elements: respect, simplicity, flexibility, integrity, communication, and professional culture. The book's easy-to-understand style makes it accessible to readers, whether they be chief nurses, nurse managers, RNS, LPNs, or nonnurse health professionals. Contributions by Nancy Valentine, Jeanette Ives Erickson, and Linda Pullins are included.

Partial Contents:

Part I: Why Use Smart Nursing? • Relationships: The Importance of a Staff-Friendly Culture • Research: Alarming Data Supporting Nursing Concerns

Part II: The Six Building Blocks of Smart Nursing • Respect: Learn to Value Nurses • Simplicity: Focus on the Basics • Flexibility: Be Adaptable • Integrity: The Foundation of Ethical Practice

Part III: Applications of Smart Nursing • Staffing: Recruiting and Retaining the Best Nurses • Teamwork: Building High Performance Teams • Safety: Preventing Medical Errors

Part IV: Looking to the Future • Benefits to Groups Outside Nursing: How CEOs, Physicians, Trustees, and Managed Care Professionals Can Help • Becoming a Lifelong Learner : Accelerate Your Professional Development • Through the Process of Change Emerges the Decade of the Nurse

Nursing Management and Leadership Series
2005   224pp   0-8261-2585-9   softcover

11 West 42nd Street, New York, NY 10036-8002 • Fax: 212-941-7842
Order Toll-Free: 877-687-7476 • Order On-line: www.springerpub.com